Preventing Patient Suicide

Clinical Assessment *and* Management

Preventing Patient Suicide

Clinical Assessment *and* Management

ROBERT I. SIMON, M.D.

Clinical Professor of Psychiatry and Director, Program in Psychiatry and Law
Georgetown University School of Medicine, Washington, D.C.
Chairman, Department of Psychiatry, Suburban Hospital,
Johns Hopkins Medicine, Bethesda, Maryland

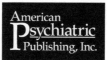

American Psychiatric Publishing, Inc.

Washington, DC
London, England

Copyright © 2011 American Psychiatric Publishing, Inc.
ALL RIGHTS RESERVED

Manufactured in the United States of America on acid-free paper
14   13   12   11   10   5   4   3   2   1
First Edition

Typeset in Adobe's Baskerville and Myriad

American Psychiatric Publishing, Inc.
1000 Wilson Boulevard
Arlington, VA 22209-3901
www.appi.org

Library of Congress Cataloging-in-Publication Data
Simon, Robert I.
    Preventing patient suicide : clinical assessment and management / by Robert I. Simon. — 1st ed.
        p. ; cm.
    Includes bibliographical references and index.
    ISBN 978-1-58562-934-3 (pbk. : alk. paper)
    1. Suicide—Prevention. 2. Suicide—Risk factors. 3. Suicidal behavior—Risk factors. I. Title.
    [DNLM: 1. Suicide—prevention & control. 2. Mental Disorders—complications. 3. Mentally Ill Persons—psychology. 4. Patients—psychology. 5. Risk Assessment—methods. WM 165]
    RC569.S557 2011
    616.85′8445--dc22

                                                          2010026853

British Library Cataloguing in Publication Data
A CIP record is available from the British Library.

*Care more for the individual patient than
for the special features of the disease.*
William Osler (1849–1919)

*This book is dedicated to all clinicians who undertake
the awesome responsibility of saving the lives of those
despairing of living.*

Contents

PART I
ASSESSMENT

Foreword

OF all the capabilities that psychiatrists (and all mental health practitioners who treat patients with diagnosable psychiatric disorders) must develop, the capacity to assess and manage suicide risk is both the most essential and the most problematic. Essential in that the clinician is in a position to effect whether the outcome is life or death, and problematic in that it has been clearly demonstrated that suicide cannot be reliably predicted in an individual, yet the psychiatrist (mental health clinician) is expected to adequately assess and manage suicide risk. In the face of this logical conundrum, Robert I. Simon, M.D., a psychiatrist with vast experience in psychiatry and the law, addresses this apparent contradiction with his discussion of the assessment and management of suicide risk in this book.

Dr. Simon confronts the problem of appropriate suicide risk assessment, as well as the legal issue of foreseeability, while at the same time reviewing up-to-date clinical research that can maximize the effectiveness of this crucial clinical assessment. He emphasizes the contemporary issues of acute versus chronic suicide risk, patients whose risk is converting from chronic to acute, and realistic clinical situations in which assessment of suicide risk is difficult, while at the same time adding his keen forensic perspective.

The author then considers management issues such as involuntary commitment and, most importantly, the management of patients who may be at high risk for suicide who do not meet local criteria for involuntary commitment—the patients we so frequently see in clinical practice. Again, a focus on chronic versus acute risk, as well as treatment-modifiable risk factors for suicide, is woven into the discussion of principles of clinical management of suicide risk.

Dr. Simon strikes a beautiful balance between the latest clinical information on suicide risk assessment and management, real clinical situations that challenge the clinician, and the inevitable forensic issues that are always present as the 800-pound gorilla in the room, as the clinician navigates in an attempt to do what's best for the patient.

Suicide prevention is the razor's edge of psychiatry. We can never know enough to be consistently successful in saving all our patients' lives—we can never be sure when we have been successful—but it is painfully obvious when we have failed in our efforts. This book is an excellent guide to doing the best we can in the most difficult of clinical situations.

Jan Fawcett, M.D.
Professor of Psychiatry
University of New Mexico School of Medicine
Albuquerque, New Mexico

Preface

PSYCHIATRISTS cannot always prevent patient suicide, even with the best of care. Nevertheless, it is a goal to be much desired. What we can do and assuredly must do is to reduce suicide risk by taking the time and making the necessary effort to know and care for the patient. This is not a radical idea. It is as old as the practice of medicine. The "know thy patient" imperative is a core theme woven throughout this book.

Knowing one's patient is not an easy task, however, given the current limitations on mental health benefits. Time is of the essence. Outpatient visits are curtailed. High-risk, acutely suicidal patients are admitted to inpatient units for short lengths of stay, some under 5 days. Stretched staffs tend to rely on suicide prevention contracts, and risk assessment checklists are commonplace. The medical record reveals many checked boxes but little documentation. Documented, competent suicide risk assessments are a rarity.

In outpatient settings, suicidal patients are often treated in split-treatment arrangements. Psychiatrists frequently see patients for brief "med checks," while therapists conduct their psychotherapy. Close collaboration is necessary to prevent the suicidal patient from "falling through the cracks." However, insurers do not pay for clinical time spent in collaboration. And e-mails and video conferencing cannot provide essential clinical data to properly assess and manage the suicidal patient.

Psychiatrists no longer have the privilege and luxury of treating patients for many months or even years. The delivery of mental health care will certainly change, though not necessarily for the better, in the years ahead. Nonetheless, psychiatrists must continue to possess a reasonable, "good enough," working knowledge of their suicidal patients in order to provide competent care, usually in close collaboration with other mental health professionals.

This book reflects my clinical experience, the shared clinical experiences of colleagues, and reliance on the evidence-based psychiatric literature. I make no claim that it sets forth a standard of care by which mental health professionals should be judged. It is written in the spirit of collegiality and with the utmost respect for clinicians who daily undertake the daunting task of assessing and managing patients at risk for suicide, and often preventing their suicide.

Robert I. Simon, M.D.

Acknowledgments

I am very grateful to Ms. Carol A. Westrick for her dedicated, diligent, and capable assistance. Without her help, this book could not have been written.

I also want to express my appreciation to Robert E. Hales, M.D., Editor-in-Chief of American Psychiatric Publishing, Inc. (APPI), for his encouragement and the opportunity to publish a book on suicide prevention. My continuing association with APPI and its excellent staff has been most gratifying. Writing a book is challenging but made easier by the support of others. Writing in isolation is a difficult, if not an impossible, task.

PART I

ASSESSMENT

CHAPTER 1

Suicide Risk Assessment

A Gateway to Treatment and Management

THE purpose of systematic suicide risk assessment is to identify modifiable and treatable risk and protective factors that inform the patient's overall treatment and management requirements (Simon 2001). Suicide risk assessment is a core competency that psychiatrists are expected to acquire during their residency (Scheiber et al. 2003). It is a gateway to the treatment and management of patients at risk for suicide.

A standard of care does not exist for the prediction of suicide (Pokorny 1983, 1993). Suicide is a rare event. Efforts to predict who will commit suicide lead to a large number of false positive and false negative predictions. No method of suicide risk assessment can reliably identify who will commit suicide (sensitivity) and who will not (specificity). Sui-

Adapted with permission from Simon RI: "Suicide Risk: Assessing the Unpredictable" in the *The American Psychiatric Publishing Textbook of Suicide Assessment and Management.* Edited by Simon RI, Hales RE. Washington, DC, American Psychiatric Publishing, 2006, pp. 1–32.

cide is the result of multiple factors, including diagnosis (psychiatric and medical), psychodynamic, genetic, familial, occupational, environmental, social, cultural, existential, and chance factors. Stressful life events have a significant association with completed suicides (Heila et al. 1999). Patients are at varying risk for suicide, and their level of risk can change rapidly. Thus, unless speaking generally, the "patient at risk for suicide" is the preferred terminology rather than the generic "suicidal patient."

Standardized suicide risk prediction scales do not identify which patient will commit suicide (Busch et al. 1993). Single scores of suicide risk assessment scales and inventories should not be relied on by clinicians as the sole basis for clinical decision making (see Chapter 10, "Suicide Risk Assessment Forms: Clinician Beware"). Structured or semi-structured suicide scales can complement, but are not a substitute for, systematic suicide risk assessment (American Psychiatric Association 2003). Malone et al. (1995) found that semi-structured screening instruments improved routine clinical assessments in the documentation and detection of lifetime suicidal behavior. Oquendo et al. (2003) have discussed the utility and limitations of research instruments in assessing suicide risk.

Self-administered suicide scales are overly sensitive and lack specificity. Suicide risk factors occur in many depressed patients who do not commit suicide. Although, occasionally, patients provide more information on a self-administered scale than in a clinical interview, patients at risk for suicide may not answer truthfully. Checklists cannot encompass all the pertinent suicide risk factors present in a given patient (Simon 2009). The plaintiff's attorney will point out the omission of pertinent suicide risk factors on the checklist used to assess the patient who later commits suicide. The standard of care does not require that specific psychological tests or checklists be used as part of the systematic assessment of suicide risk (Bongar et al. 1992; see Chapter 11, "Imminent Suicide, Passive Suicidal Ideation, and Other Intractable Myths").

Actuarial analysis reveals that most depressed patients do not kill themselves. For instance, the 2002 national suicide rate in the general population was 11.1 per 100,000 per year (Heron et al. 2009). The suicide rate or absolute risk of suicide for individuals with bipolar and other mood disorders is estimated to be 193 per 100,000, or a relative risk of 18 times that of the general population (Baldessarini 2003). Thus, 99,807 patients with these disorders will not commit suicide in a single year. The same actuarial analysis can be applied to other psychiatric disorders. The suicide rate for schizophrenia, alcohol, and drug abuse is also 18 times the 2002 national suicide rate. On an actuarial basis alone, the vast majority of patients will not commit suicide. Actuarial analysis, however, is more useful in identifying diagnostic groups at higher risk than in trying to predict the suicide of a specific patient (Addy 1992). Actuarial analysis does not identify specific treatable risk and modifiable protective factors. The clinical challenge is to identify those patients with depression at high *risk* for suicide at any given time (Jacobs et al. 1999).

The standard of care does require that psychiatrists and other mental health professionals adequately assess suicide risk when it is indicated. Risk assessments that systematically evaluate both risk and protective factors (see Figure 1–1 later in this chapter) should meet any reasonable definition of "adequate." Conceptually, it is a process of analysis and synthesis that identifies, prioritizes, and integrates acute and chronic risk and protective factors. Suicide risk assessment, based on current research that identifies risk and protective factors for suicide, enables the clinician to make evidence-based treatment and safety management decisions (Fawcett et al. 1987; Linehan et al. 1983).

Professional organizations recognize the need for developing evidence-based and clinical consensus recommendations to be applied to the management of various diseases, including such behavioral states as suicide (Simon 2002; Taylor 2010). The American Academy of Child and Adolescent Psychiatry has published "Practice Parameter for the Assessment and Treatment of Children and Adolescents With Suicidal Behavior" (Shaffer et al. 1997). Also, the American Psychiatric Association Work Group on Suicidal Behavior has developed a practice guideline for the assessment and treatment of patients with suicidal behaviors (American Psychiatric Association 2003).

Case Example

A 32-year-old single woman who works as a computer specialist is brought to an urban community hospital department after impulsively ingesting an unknown quantity of aspirin tablets and then slashing her arms with a knife. She is severely agitated, responding to command hallucinations to kill herself. The patient became acutely depressed and agitated following the break-up of a brief relationship, her first "serious" intimate relationship. At age 16 years, the patient made a few superficial scratches on her wrist with a razor, following a "disappointment" with a young person she idolized from afar. During the week prior to admission, she abused alcohol and methamphetamine.

An admission drug screen is positive for these substances. The salicylate level is markedly elevated.

Upon admission to the psychiatric unit, the patient is placed on one-to-one safety management. Her agitation and aggressive-impulsive behaviors require placement in open-door seclusion with an attendant sitting by the door. Nursing staff protocol requires that all patients be encouraged to verbally agree with or sign a suicide prevention contract. The patient does not understand the purpose of the contract. Nevertheless, she signs the contract. Psychiatric examination reveals a thought disorder, severe agitation, bizarre facial grimaces and mannerisms, confusion, hopelessness, command hallucinations, flat affect, insomnia, and inability to interact with the psychiatrist, unit staff, and other patients.

The psychiatrist and the psychiatric unit's social worker speak with the patient's mother and siblings at the time of admission. The psychiatrist relies on the emergency exception to consent in speaking to family members without the patient's authorization. He learns that the patient's parents were divorced when she was 7 years old. She sees her father infrequently. The patient has a close relationship with her mother, older brother, and younger sister.

There is no history of physical or sexual abuse. The mother reveals that her daughter was a good student, excelling in mathematics. Her relationship with coworkers is good. However, she has had few friends. The patient holds strong religious beliefs. She is described by her siblings as creative, artistic, and a loner. In the past, the patient has reacted to major disappointments with depression and suicidal thoughts, sometimes accompanied by "strange" facial movements and grimaces. The family history is positive for mental illness. A paternal uncle, diagnosed as a "manic-depressive," committed suicide with a shotgun 10 years ago. A reclusive maternal aunt has been diagnosed as a "chronic schizophrenic."

The patient is living at home. The psychiatrist asks about guns in the home. The patient's brother states that there is a shotgun at home used for skeet shooting. The brother agrees to remove the gun from the home. A follow-up call by the social worker confirms that the gun was removed from the home and secured in a safe place. The psychiatrist's systematic suicide risk assessment of the patient on admission is rated as high (see Figure 1–2 later in this chapter).

The psychiatrist makes a diagnosis of schizophrenia, disorganized type, and substance abuse (alcohol and methamphetamine). He prescribes an atypical antipsychotic medication, a benzodiazepine, for control of severe agitation, and a sleep medication. The psychiatrist will consider a suicide reduction drug, such as clozapine for patients with schizophrenia, if suicide ideation does not remit. In his initial suicide risk assessment, the psychiatrist evaluates both acute and chronic risk factors as well as current protective factors. He continues to assess the patient's acute suicide risk factors over the course of the hospitalization.

On the day after admission, the patient is less agitated. She does not require seclusion. On the third hospital day, command hallucinations are indistinct. The patient is more communicative with the hospital staff and other patients. By the fifth hospital day, the patient states the command hallucinations "have gone away." She is not agitated. Suicidal ideation continues but without intent or plan. The patient's bizarre facial grimaces and mannerisms observed on admission are no longer present. Hopelessness and confusion diminish.

The patient attends all the assigned group therapies. She benefits from individual and group supportive therapies. The patient develops a therapeutic alliance with the psychiatrist and the treatment team. Her affect, however, remains flat. Her thought processes are logical, but abstracting ability for proverbs is impaired. Mild insomnia is present. Concentration is poor. The patient willingly takes her medication, though she experiences mild to moderate side effects.

Utilizing evidence-based studies, the psychiatrist assesses the risk factors associated with an increased risk of suicide in schizophrenic patients. These include a previous suicide attempt (robust "predictor" of eventual completed suicide), substance abuse, depressive symptoms, especially hopelessness, male sex, early stage in illness, good premorbid history and intellectual functioning, and frequent exacerbations and remissions (Meltzer 2001). The psychiatrist has read the International Clozaril/Leponex Suicide Prevention Trial (InterSePT) study, which indicated significant risk factors for suicide in schizophrenic patients to include the diagnosis of schizoaffective disorder, current or lifetime alcohol/substance abuse or smoking, hospitalization in the previous 3 years to prevent a suicide attempt, and the number of lifetime suicide attempts (Meltzer et al. 2003a).

A systematic suicide risk assessment is performed on hospital day 6 (see Figure 1–3 later in this chapter) and is compared with the admission suicide risk assessment (see Figure 1–2 later in this chapter). Although most of the acute psychotic symptoms have improved or remitted, suicidal ideation continues. The overall risk of suicide is assessed at "moderate" on day 6. The psychiatrist determines that the patient needs an additional week of inpatient treatment. Because of the patient's overall improvement, the insurer authorizes coverage for 2 additional days after a doctor-to-doctor appeal. The psychiatrist's experience indicates that most patients at moderate suicide risk can be treated as outpatients. The psychiatrist crafts an outpatient treatment plan based on the patient's clinical and safety needs. He understands that the decision to discharge a patient is the psychiatrist's responsibility. The psychiatrist's decision is not based on the insurer's denial of benefits. An insurer's denial of benefits is not considered an acceptable justification for placing the patient at increased risk for suicide.

The patient's postdischarge plan recommends once-per-week supportive psychotherapy and medication management with the psychiatrist. The patient is also referred to the hospital's partial hospitalization and substance abuse programs, which she will attend the day after discharge. The patient is eager to return to work but agrees to remain on sick leave for another 3 weeks. She recognizes the importance of adhering to the follow-up care plan. The patient plans to pursue her artistic interests. Her mother and siblings are very supportive, which is a major protective factor. The psychiatrist assesses other protective factors, including the patient's ability to form a therapeutic alliance, adherence to treatment, treatment benefit, strong religious values, positive reasons for living, and commitment to the follow-up care plan. The psychiatrist's discharge diagnosis is schizophrenia, single episode, in partial remission, and substance abuse disorder (alcohol and methamphetamine).

Standard of Care

Each state defines the standard of care required of physicians. For example, in *Stepakoff v. Kantar* (1985), a suicide case, the standard applied by the court was the "duty to exercise that degree of skill and care ordinarily employed in similar circumstances by other psychiatrists." The duty of care established by the court was that of the "average psychiatrist." In an increasing number of states, the standard of care is that of the "reasonable, prudent practitioner" (Peters 2000). The legal standard must be distinguished from the professional standard of "best practices" (Simon 2005).

In a suicide case, the courts evaluate the psychiatrist's management of the patient who attempted or committed suicide to determine whether the suicide risk assessment process was reasonable and the patient's attempt or suicide was foreseeable. An "imperfect fit," however, exists between medical and legal terminology. *Foreseeability* is a legal term of art. It is a commonsense, probabilistic concept, not a scientific construct. Foreseeability is defined as the reasonable anticipation that harm or injury is likely to result from certain acts or omissions (Black 1999). Foreseeability is not the same as predicting when a patient will attempt or commit suicide. It should not be confused with predictability, for which no professional standard exists. Foreseeability must also be distinguished from preventability. A patient's suicide may be preventable in hindsight, but it was not foreseeable at the time of assessment.

Only the risk of suicide is determinable. The prediction of suicide is opaque, but there is reasonable visibility for assessing suicide risk. When contemporaneously documented, systematic suicide risk assessments help provide the court with guidance. When suicide risk assessments are not performed or documented, the court is less able to evaluate the clinical complexities and ambiguities that exist in the assessment, treatment, and management of patients at risk for suicide. In malpractice litigation, the failure to perform an adequate suicide risk assessment is often alleged along with other claims of negligence. It is rarely asserted as the only complaint (Simon 2004).

Systematic Suicide Risk Assessment

Systematic suicide risk assessment identifies acute, modifiable, and treatable risk and protective factors essential to informing the psychiatrist's treatment and safety management of patients at risk for suicide (see Figure 1–1 later in this chapter). It is easy to overlook important risk and protective factors in the absence of systematic assessment. Systematic suicide assessment helps the clinician gather important information and piece together risk factors with which to construct a clinical mosaic of the suicidal patient.

Suicide risk assessment is an integral part of the psychiatric examination, yet it is rarely performed systematically or, when performed, it is not contemporaneously documented. Risk and protective factors may be noted but without any analysis or synthesis. It is evident from the review of quality assurance records and the forensic analysis of suicide cases in litigation that the extent of suicide risk assessment usually is no more than "Patient denies HI, SI, CFS" (homicidal ideation, suicidal ideation, contracts for safety). Frequently, one finds no documentation of suicide risk assessment or only the statement that the "patient denies suicidal ideation." Suicide risk assessment is a core clinical skill that informs the treatment and management of patients at risk for suicide (Simon 2001). Often, a talismanic "no-harm contract" replaces performing an adequate suicide risk assessment. Laypersons could just as easily ask these same questions and obtain a no-harm contract. Moreover, there is no evidence that suicide safety contracts decrease or prevent suicide (Stanford et al. 1994). The road to patient suicides is often strewn with safety contracts. In the case example presented earlier in this chapter, systematic suicide risk assessment supplants a reliance on a suicide prevention contract.

Why so many psychiatrists, sued or not sued, fail to perform and document adequate suicide risk assessments is discussed elsewhere (see Chapter 12, "Quality Assurance Review of Suicide Risk Assessments: Reality and Remedy")? In inpatient settings, short lengths of stay and the rapid turnover of seriously ill patients may distract the clinician from performing adequate risk assessments. Also, the focus of clinical attention rapidly shifts away from knowing the patient to pressing discharge planning.

Approximately 25% of patients at risk for suicide do not admit having suicidal ideation to the clinician but do tell their families (Robins 1981). Hall et al. (1999) found that 69 of 100 patients had had only fleeting or no suicidal thoughts before they made a suicide attempt. None of these patients reported having had a specific plan before his or her impulsive suicide attempt. Also, because this was the first attempt for 67% of these patients, a prior suicide attempt did not exist.

Patients who are determined to commit suicide regard the psychiatrist and other mental health professionals as the enemy (Resnick 2002). Just asking the patient at risk for suicide about the presence of suicidal ideation, suicide intent, and a suicide plan and receiving a denial cannot be relied on by itself. If possible, family members or others who know the patient should be consulted. Even when the patient is telling the truth, it is unwise to equate the patient's denial of suicidal ideation with an absence of suicide risk.

The Principles of Medical Ethics With Annotations Especially Applicable to Psychiatry (American Psychiatric Association 2001) includes the following statement: "Psychiatrists at times may find it necessary, in order to protect the patient or community from imminent danger, to reveal confidential information disclosed by the patient" (Section 4, Annotation 8). Management of patients at high risk for suicide may require the breaking of patient confidence and involvement of the family or significant others (e.g., to obtain vital information, to administer and monitor medications, to remove lethal weapons, to assist in hospitalization). Statutory waiver of confidential information is provided in some states when a patient seriously threatens self-harm (Simon 1992, p. 269). If the severely disturbed patient lacks the mental capacity to consent, a substitute health care decision-maker should be interviewed. In a number of states, proxy consent by next of kin is not permitted for patients with mental illnesses. If an emergency exists, the emergency exception to patient consent may be invoked (Simon and Shuman 2007). Just listening to others without divulg-

---

TABLE 1–1. Suicide risk assessment data gathering: hospital admission

---

- Identify distinctive individual suicide risk factors.
- Identify acute suicide risk factors.
- Identify protective factors.
- Evaluate medical history and laboratory studies.
- Obtain treatment team information.
- Interview patient's significant others.
- Speak with current or prior treaters.
- Review the patient's current and prior hospital records.

Note. Modify for outpatient use.
Source. Adapted from Simon RI: "Suicide Risk Assessment in Managed Care Settings." *Primary Psychiatry* 7:42–43, 46–49, 2002. Used with permission.

---

ing information about the patient does not violate confidentiality unless the patient withholds consent for any contact with others. It may be possible to speak with others once a therapeutic alliance develops and the patient consents. The Health Insurance Portability and Accountability Act of 1996 (HIPAA) permits psychiatrists and other health care providers who are treating the same patient to communicate without expressed permission from the patient (45 Code of Federal Regulations § 164.502).

Observational information obtained from the psychiatric examination may provide objective information about suicide risk factors, thus avoiding total reliance on the patient's reporting (see Chapter 4, "Behavioral Risk Assessment of the Guarded Suicidal Patient"). For example, slash marks on the arms or neck, or burns or other wounds, may be apparent. The mental status examination may reveal diminished concentration, bizarre ideation, evidence of command hallucinations, incapacity to cooperate, restlessness, agitation, severe thought disorder, impulsivity, and alcohol or drug withdrawal symptoms. The degree of irritability can be rapidly assessed in patients with major depressive disorder and is correlated with depression severity and suicide attempts (Perlis et al. 2005).

Suicide risk assessment bears an analogy to weather forecasting (Monahan and Steadman 1996; Simon 1992). Determining the clinician's level of confidence in the available patient data is essential for the treatment and management of suicide risk. Table 1–1 contains a suicide risk assessment approach for data gathering that can be used by the clinician. The standard of care requires that the clinician gather sufficient information upon which to base an adequate suicide risk assessment. The assessment approach can alert the clinician to deficiencies in the data collection.

Systematic risk assessment itself is an impetus to gather essential clinical information about the patient. It reminds the clinician to consider multiple data sources. When the clinical situation turns stormy, clinicians, like pilots, must rely on their instruments. Systematic suicide risk assessment is that instrument in managing the suicidal patient.

Suicide Risk Factors

General risk factors such as a recent suicide attempt, hopelessness, or family history of suicide apply across most clinical settings. Individual suicide risk factors are unique and specific to the patient. The stuttering patient who no longer stutters when suicidal is a classic example. Suicide risk factors can be culturally determined, as is the case with shame suicides in certain Far East cultures. Suicide risk factors occur under certain circumstances, as when individuals are jailed for the first time. Age-related contagion effect is an important suicide risk factor for adolescents who have been directly exposed to a completed peer suicide. Although clinicians rely mostly on general suicide risk factors, individual, cultural, and contextual risk factors must also be considered.

There is no pathognomonic risk factor for suicide. A single suicide risk factor does not have adequate statistical power on which to base an assessment. Suicide risk assessment cannot be predicated on the basis of any one factor (Meltzer et al. 2003b); the assessment of suicide risk is multifactorial. Moreover, a number of retrospective community-based psychological autopsies and studies of psychiatric patients who have committed suicide have identified general risk factors (Fawcett et al. 1993). Evidence-based general risk factors are applied to the clinical presentations of individual patients in concert with their unique risk factors.

Short-term suicide risk factors derived from a prospective study of patients with major affective disorders were statistically significant within 1 year of assessment (Fawcett et al. 1990). Short-term risk factors included panic attacks, psychic anxiety, loss of pleasure and interest, moderate alcohol abuse, depressive turmoil (mixed states), diminished concentration, and global insomnia. Short-term risk factors were predominantly severe, anxiety driven, and treatable by a variety of psychotropic drugs (Fawcett 2001).

Suicidal ideation is a key risk factor. In the National Comorbidity Survey, the transition probabilities from suicide ideation to suicide plan were 34% and from a plan to attempt were 72% (Kessler et al. 1999). The probability of transition from suicidal ideation to an unplanned suicide attempt was 26%. In this study, approximately 90% of unplanned and 60% of planned first attempts occurred within 1 year of the onset of suicidal ideation. Systematic suicide risk assessment should be performed when the patient reports passive suicidal ideations (e.g., "I hope God takes me" vs. "I'm going to kill myself"). Passive ideation can become quickly active. Also, the patient may be minimizing or hiding active suicide ideation. In passive suicidal ideation, the intent is to die by indirect means (see Chapter 11, "Imminent Suicide, Passive Suicidal Ideation, and Other Intractable Myths").

When evaluating a patient's suicidal ideation, the clinician should consider specific content, intensity, duration, and prior episodes. Mann et al. (1999) found that the severity of an individual's ideation is an indicator of risk for attempting suicide. Beck et al. (1990) determined that when patients were asked about suicidal ideation at its worst point, patients with high scores were 14 times more likely to commit suicide compared with patients having low scores.

Patients with major depression and generalized anxiety disorder have higher levels of suicidal ideation when compared with depressed patients who do not have generalized anxiety disorder (Zimmerman and Chelminski 2003). Comorbid anxiety and depression occur in over 50% of persons with nonbipolar major depressive disorders (Zimmerman et al. 2002). The combination of severe depression and anxiety or panic attacks can prove lethal. A patient may be able to tolerate depression. When anxiety or panic is also present, the patient's life may become unbearable, dangerously elevating suicide risk. Anxiety (agitation) symptoms should be treated aggressively while antidepressant medications are being given an opportunity to work. Many patients demonstrate a significant antidepressant response within the first 1–2 weeks of treatment (Posternak et al. 2005).

Time is on the side of patients at risk for suicide who are treated rapidly and effectively. For example, in patients with severe depression, time works against them when treatment is delayed or ineffective. The mental disorder often progresses and becomes entrenched. Secondary effects, such as work impairment and disrupted relationships, lead to despair, demoralization, and an increased risk of suicide. Suicide reduction medications, such as lithium and clozapine, should be considered for bipolar and schizophrenia patients, respectively (Baldessarini et al. 2006).

Long-term suicide risk factors in patients with major affective disorder are associated with suicides completed 2–10 years following assessment (Fawcett et al. 1990). Information about long-term suicide risk factors is derived from community-based psychological autopsies and the retrospective study of psychiatric patients who have committed suicide (Fawcett et al. 1993). Long-term suicide risk factors include suicidal ideation, suicidal intent, severe hopelessness, and prior attempts. Suicide risk increases with the total number of risk factors, providing a quasi-quantitative dimension to suicide risk assessment (Murphy et al. 1992).

Patients from diagnostic groups such as major affective disorders, chronic alcoholism and substance abuse, schizophrenia, and borderline personality disorder are at increased risk for suicide (Fawcett et al. 1993). Roose et al. (1983) found that delusional depressed patients were five times more likely to commit suicide than depressed patients who were not delusional. Busch et al. (2003) also indicated that there was an association between psychosis and suicide in 54% of the 76 inpatient suicides. In the Collaborative Study of Depression (Fawcett et al. 1987), no significant difference in suicide rate was shown between depressed and delusionally depressed patients. Patients that had delusions of thought insertion, grandeur, and mind reading, however, were significantly represented in the suicide group (Fawcett et al. 1987). Numerous follow-up studies have not indicated that patients with psychotic depression are more likely to commit suicide than patients with nonpsychotic depression (Coryell et al. 2003; Vythilingam et al. 2003). Recent research indicates that suicide risk increases with the severity of psychosis (Warman et al. 2004). Electroconvulsive therapy may produce rapid reduction of suicide risk in severely depressed patients whose symptoms failed to respond to adequate drug trials.

Patients often display distinctive, individual suicide risk and preventive factor patterns. Suicide patterns may be identified from prior exacerbations of suicidal ideation, suicidal crises, or actual attempts. Understanding a patient's psychodynamics and psychological responses to past and current life stressors is important. In the case example presented earlier in this chapter, when the patient was depressed and at risk for suicide, she displayed bizarre facial mannerisms. Some unusual prodromal suicide risk factors can emerge when the patient becomes suicidal; for example, the stuttering patient whose speech clears, the patient who compulsively whistles, and the patient who self-inflicts facial excoriations. Most patients experience more common suicide risk patterns, such as suicidal ideation, within a few hours or days following the onset of early morning awakening. Knowing a patient's distinctive, prodromal suicide risk factors along with his or her psychodynamics is very helpful in treatment and safety management. Strongly held values, such as religious beliefs, and reasons for living can be significant protective factors.

Demographic suicide risk factors include, for example, age, gender, race, and marital status. The suicide rates for white males over age 65 years are elevated. White males over age 85 years have the highest suicide rates. Males commit suicide at a rate three to four times greater than that of females. Females make suicide attempts at a rate three to four times greater than that of men. Divorced individuals are at significantly increased risk for suicide compared with married individuals. The suicide rate is higher among white individuals (with the exception of young adults) than among African Americans. Demographic suicide risk factors, though significant, only serve to supplement the assessment of individual risk factors.

A family history of mental illness, especially of suicide, is a significant suicide risk factor. A genetic component exists in the etiology of affective disorders, schizophrenia, alcoholism and substance abuse, and cluster B personality disorders. These psychiatric disorders are associated with most suicides (Mann and Arango 1999). Genetic and familial transmission of suicide risk is independent of the transmission of psychiatric illnesses (Brent et al. 1996). Psychiatric illnesses are a necessary but not necessarily sufficient cause of patient suicides. Patients with intractable, malignant psychiatric disorders that end in suicide often have strong genetic and familial components to their illnesses.

In schizophrenia, the completed lifetime suicide rate is 9%–13%. The estimated number of suicides annually in the United States among patients with schizophrenia is 3,600 (12% of total suicides). The lifetime suicide attempt rate is 20%–40%. Suicide is the leading cause of death among persons with schizophrenia who are younger than age 35 years. Suicide is a risk in schizophrenia throughout the individual's life cycle (Heila et al. 1997; Meltzer and Okaly 1995); however, suicide tends to occur in the early stages of illness and during an active phase (Meltzer 2001).

In the case example presented earlier in this chapter, the patient's suicide attempt is directed by command hallucinations. The earlier psychiatric literature indicated that command hallucinations accounted for relatively few suicides in patients with schizophrenia (Breier and Astrachan 1984; Roy 1982). Nonetheless, an auditory hallucination that commands suicide is an important risk factor, which requires careful assessment. The patient needs to be asked: "Are the auditory hallucinations that are commanding suicide acute or chronic, syntonic or dystonic, familiar or unfamiliar voices?" It is important to find out if the patient is able to resist the hallucinatory commands or if the patient has attempted suicide in obedience to the voices.

Junginger (1990) reported that 39% of patients with command hallucinations obeyed them. Patients were more likely to comply with hallucinatory commands if they could identify the voices. Kasper et al. (1996) found that 84% of psychiatric inpatients with command hallucinations had obeyed them within the past 30 days. The resistance to command hallucinations that dictate dangerous acts appears to be greater than the resistance to commands to perform nondangerous acts (Juninger 1995). This is not as true for patients who have obeyed command hallucinations dictating self-destructive behaviors. In a study of command hallucinations for suicide, 80% of suicide attempters reported having made at least one attempt in response to command hallucinations (Harkavy-Friedman et al. 2003). Hellerstein et al. (1987) studied the content of command hallucinations and grouped them in the following categories: 52% suicide, 14% nonviolent acts, 12% nonlethal injury to self or others, 5% homicide, and 17% unspecified. Thus, 69% of command hallucinations dictated violence. Patients with auditory hallucinations that command suicide should be presumptively assessed at high risk for suicide, requiring immediate psychiatric treatment and management.

Harris and Barraclough (1997) abstracted 249 reports from the medical literature regarding the mortality of mental disorders. They compared observed numbers of suicides in individuals with mental disorders with those expected in the general population. The standardized mortality ratio (SMR)—a measure of the relative risk of suicide for a particular disorder compared with the expected rate in the general population (SMR of 1)—was calculated for each disorder by dividing observed mortality by expected mortality. The authors concluded, "If these results can be generalized, then virtually all mental disorders have an increased risk for suicide excepting mental retardation and dementia."

Harris and Barraclough also calculated the SMR for all psychiatric diagnoses by the treatment setting. The SMR for inpatients was 5.82, and for outpatients was 18.09. Prior suicide attempts by any method had the highest SMR, 38.36. Suicide risk was highest in the 2 years following the first attempt. A correct diagnosis is essential. The SMR for psychiatric, neurological, and medical disorders can be helpful to the psychiatrist in assessing the risk of suicide for a specific diagnosis.

Baldessarini (2003) and colleagues found that the overall SMR for bipolar disorder was 21.8. The SMR was 1.4 times higher for women than for men. Most suicide acts occur within the first 5 years after the onset of illness. The SMR for bipolar II disorder was 24.1, compared with an SMR of 17.0 for bipolar I disorder and 11.8 for unipolar depression.

The finding of a high SMR for prior suicide attempts is supported by other studies (Fawcett 2001). Between 7%–12% of patients who make suicide attempts commit suicide within 10 years, thus making it a significant chronic risk factor for suicide. The risk of completed suicide is highest during the first year after the attempt. Suicide rehearsals, behavioral or mental, are common. Recent near-lethal attempts are frequently followed within days by a completed suicide. Most suicides, however, occur in patients with no history of prior attempts. The majority of patients who committed suicide had not communicated their suicide intent during their last appointment (Isometsa et al. 1995). In a retrospective study of 76 inpatient suicides, Busch et al. (2003) found that 77% of the patients denied suicidal ideation as their last recorded communication. Mann et al. (1999) found that prior suicide attempts and hopelessness are the most powerful clinical "predictors" of completed suicide. The rate of suicide completion during first attempts is high, especially among males (62%; females, 38%) (Isometsa and Lonnqvist 1998). Previous attempters (82%) used at least two different methods in attempts and completed suicides.

Research indicates that high risk factors associated with attempted suicide in adults are depression, prior suicide attempt(s), hopelessness, suicidal ideation, alcohol abuse, cocaine use, and recent loss of an important relationship (Murphy et al. 1992). In youths, the strongest factors associated with suicide attempts are depression, alcohol or other drug use disorder, and aggressive or disruptive behaviors. Weisman and Worden (1972) devised a risk-rescue rating in suicide assessment as a descriptive and quantitative method of determining the lethality of suicide attempt.

Populations at Risk for Suicide

Practice parameters exist for the assessment and treatment of children and adolescents with suicidal behavior (Shaffer et al. 1997). Risk factors for adolescents include prior attempts, affective disorder, substance abuse, living alone, male gender, age 16 years or older, and a history of physical and/or sexual abuse. Adverse childhood experiences—for example, emotional, physical, and sexual abuse—are associated with an increased risk of attempted suicide throughout the lifespan (Dube et al. 2001). More suicidal women than suicidal men have experienced childhood abuse (Kaplan et al. 1995). Brent (2001) provides a framework for the assessment of suicide risk in the adolescent that can be used to determine immediate disposition, intensity of treatment, and level of care.

In adults over age 65 years, important correlates of late-life suicide are depression, physical illnesses, functional impairment, personality traits of neuroticism, social isolation, and loss of important relationships (Conwell and Duberstein 2001). The suicide rate for men 85 years and older is substantially higher (60 per 100,000) (Loebel 2005). Affective disorder is the risk factor with the strongest correlation. Among older adults, 41% saw their primary care physician within 28 days of committing suicide (Isometsa et al. 1995). Thus, primary care is an important point of suicide prevention for elders at high risk.

Personality disorders place a patient at increased risk for suicide (Linehan et al. 2000). The risk for suicide is 7 times greater in patients with personality disorders than in the general population (Harris and Barraclough 1997). Among patients who commit suicide, 30%–40% have personality disorders (Bronisch 1996; Duberstein and Conwell 1997). Cluster B personality disorders, particularly borderline and antisocial personality disorders, place patients at increased risk for suicide (Duberstein and Conwell 1997). The presence of personality disorders, when comorbid with bipolar disorder, is an independent suicide risk factor that increases lifetime risk of suicide (Garno et al. 2005). In patients with borderline personality disorder, impulsivity was associated with a high number of suicide attempts, after substance abuse and a lifetime diagnosis of depressive disorder were controlled for (Brodsky et al. 1997). In a longitudinal study of personality disorder, a combination of borderline personality disorder, major affective disorder, and alcoholism was found in a fatal subgroup (Stone 1993).

Personality disorder, negative recent life events, and Axis I comorbidity were identified in a large sample of patients who committed suicide (Heikkinen et al. 1997). Recent stressful life events, including workplace difficulties, family problems, unemployment, and financial trouble, were highly represented among patients with personality disorders. Personality disorders and comorbidity of other factors, such as depressive symptoms and substance abuse disorders, are frequently found among patients who commit suicide (Isometsa et al. 1996; Suominen et al. 2000).

Gunderson and Ridolfi (2002) estimated that suicide threats and gestures occur repeatedly in 90% of patients with borderline personality disorder. With the borderline patient, the clinician's suicide risk assessment should pay special attention to comorbidity, especially mood disorder, substance abuse, prior suicide attempts or self-mutilating behaviors, impulsivity, and unpleasant recent-life events. Self-mutilating behaviors that commonly occur in borderline patients include cutting (80%), bruising (34%), burning (20%), head banging (15%), and biting (7%).

Although self-mutilation is considered to be parasuicidal behavior (without lethal intent), the risk of suicide is doubled when self-mutilation is present (Stone 1987). Retrospectively, it may be difficult or impossible to distinguish a nonlethal suicide gesture from an actual suicide attempt. *Suicidal intent* is defined as the subjective expectation and desire to die by a self-destructive act (American Psychiatric Association 2003). For example, the clinician must consider intent, not just behavior. A patient takes 10 aspirin tablets in the belief that it will result in death. A patient taking 6 mg/day of a benzodiazepine who overdoses on 180 1-mg tablets may not have any intention to commit suicide and knows that death will not likely occur. An *aborted attempt* occurs when the intent to harm is interrupted and no physical harm results. *Lethality* refers to the danger to life by a suicide method or act. O'Carroll et al. (1996) provide definitions for a variety of suicidal behaviors.

Psychiatrists have difficulty gauging the imminence of suicide. No suicide risk factor(s) identifies imminence. Imminence defies definition; it is not a medical or psychiatric term. Imminence is another word for prediction. The patient who points a loaded gun at his or her head or is perched on a bridge is a high-risk psychiatric emergency. But individuals have been "talked out" of pulling the trigger or jumping. Persons intent on committing suicide are usually ambivalent until the last moment. Suicide risk is in constant flux. It is imperative to identify, treat, and manage the patient's acute risk factors that are driving a suicide crisis than to undertake the impossible task of trying to predict whether or when a suicide attempt may occur. Imminent suicide creates the illusion of short-term prediction (see Chapter 11, "Imminent Suicide, Passive Suicidal Ideation, and Other Intractable Myths").

Impulsivity, a trait factor or predisposition usually associated with alcohol and substance abuse, is an important suicide risk factor requiring careful assessment (Moeller et al. 2001). Impulsivity also has been found in many suicide attempters with major depressive disorder, panic disorder, and aggressive behaviors linked to the serotonergic system (Pezawas et al. 2002). Simon et al. (2001), in a case-control study of 153 case subjects, found that 24% of the subjects spent less than 5 minutes between the decision to attempt suicide and a near-lethal attempt.

Patients who harm themselves are more impulsive than the general population. Patients who repeatedly harm themselves are found to be more impulsive than patients who harm themselves for the first time (Evans et al. 1996). Impulsivity can be both acute and chronic. A history of chronic impulsivity can become acute when heightened by life stress, loss, and anxiety. Suicide attempts or violent suicide may often result (Fawcett 2001). Mann et al. (1999) found that suicide attempters with major depressive disorder have higher levels of aggression and impulsivity than nonattempters.

Impulsivity/aggression can be assessed clinically by asking the patient questions about violent rages, assaultive behaviors, arrests, destruction of property, spending sprees, speeding tickets, sexual indiscretions, hostility, easy provocation, and other indicia of poor impulse control (McGirr et al. 2009). A history of impulsive, aggressive behaviors toward self or others is a chronic risk factor for suicide (Brent and Mann 2005).

"Shame suicides" can occur in individuals faced with intolerable humiliation (e.g., scandal, criminal charges). A "shame suicide" may be an impulsive act in a narcissistically vulnerable person. However, it may not be associated with a diagnosable mental disorder (Roy 1986).

A patient's suicide risk may be exacerbated by problems caused by the treater. Examples include cases in which the treater causes physical or psychological impairment, exploits the patient, or displays incompetence, indifference, negative countertransference, fatigue ("burnout"), or deficient language skills (Simon and Gutheil 2004). To perform an adequate suicide risk assessment, the clinician must be able to understand idiomatic phrases and slang expressions. In one instance, a severely depressed, suicidal patient with opioid dependence told the psychiatrist that she had "gone cold turkey." The psychiatrist, having limited English language skills, proceeded to ask the patient if she had an eating disorder.

Suicide Risk Assessment Methodology

A number of suicide risk assessment models are available to the clinician (Beck et al. 1998; Clark and Fawcett 1999; Jacobs et al. 1999; Linehan 1993; Mays 2004; Rudd et al. 2001; Shea 2004). Only a few methods can be cited here. No suicide risk assessment model has been empirically tested for reliability and validity (Busch et al. 1993). Clinicians can also develop their own systematic risk assessment methods based on their training, clinical experience, and familiarity with the evidence-based psychiatric literature. The example of suicide risk assessment illustrated in Figures 1–1, 1–2, and 1–3 represents just one way of *conceptualizing* systematic assessment. The model in Figure 1–1 is a *teaching tool* designed to encourage a systematic approach to suicide risk assessment. It should not be used as a form or protocol to be applied in a robotic fashion. The use of stand-alone suicide risk assessment forms is not recommended.

Suicide risk factors vary in number and importance according to the individual patient. The clinician's reasoned judgment is central in identifying and assigning clinical weight to risk and protective factors. A common error is to omit assessment of protective factors along with risk factors. It is important to assess protective factors against suicide to achieve a balanced assessment of suicide risk. As noted previously, each patient has a distinctive suicide risk factor profile that should receive a high priority for identification and assessment. Protective factors tend to be more variable. The risk factor profile or prodrome tends to recur during a subsequent psychiatric illness.

Assessment factors[a]	Risk	Protective
Individual		
Distinctive clinical features (prodrome)		
Religious beliefs		
Reasons for living		
Clinical		
Current attempt (lethality)		
Therapeutic alliance		
Treatment adherence		
Treatment benefit		
Suicidal ideation		
Suicide intent		
Suicide plan		
Hopelessness		
Prior attempts (lethality)		
Panic attacks		
Psychic anxiety		
Loss of pleasure and interest		
Alcohol/drug abuse		
Depressive turmoil (mixed states)		
Diminished concentration		
Global insomnia		
Psychiatric diagnoses (Axis I and Axis II)		
Symptom severity		
Comorbidity		
Recent discharge from psychiatric hospital		
Impulsivity/aggression		

FIGURE 1–1. Systematic suicide risk assessment: a conceptual model.

Assessment factors[a]	Risk	Protective
Clinical *(continued)*		
Agitation (akathisia)		
Physical illness		
Family history of mental illness (suicide)		
Childhood sexual/physical abuse		
Mental competency		
Interpersonal Relations		
Work or school		
Family		
Spousal or partner		
Children		
Situational		
Living circumstances		
Employment or school status		
Availability of guns		
Managed care setting		
Demographic		
Age		
Gender		
Marital status		
Race/ethnicity		
Overall risk ratings[b]		

FIGURE 1–1. Systematic suicide risk assessment: a conceptual model *(continued).*

[a]Rate risk and protective factors present as low (L), moderate (M), high (H), nonfactor (O), or range (e.g., L–M, M–H).
[b]Judge overall suicide risk as low, moderate, high, or a range of risk.
Source. Adapted with permission from Simon 2004.

Assessment factors[a]	Risk	Protective
Individual		
Distinctive clinical features (prodrome)	H	
Religious beliefs	O	
Reasons for living	O	
Clinical		
Current attempt (lethality)	H	
Therapeutic alliance	H	
Treatment adherence	L	
Treatment benefit	O	
Suicidal ideation (command hallucinations)	H	
Suicide intent	H	
Suicide plan	O	
Hopelessness	M–H	
Prior attempts (lethality)	L	
Panic attacks	O	
Psychic anxiety	O	
Loss of pleasure and interest	H	
Alcohol/drug abuse	H	
Depressive turmoil (mixed states)	O	
Diminished concentration	H	
Global insomnia	M–H	
Psychiatric diagnoses (Axis I and Axis II)	H	
Symptom severity	H	
Comorbidity	H	
Recent discharge from psychiatric hospital (within 3 months)	O	
Impulsivity/aggression	M–H	
Agitation (akathisia)	H	

FIGURE 1–2. Admission systematic suicide risk assessment: case example.

Assessment factors[a]	Risk	Protective
Clinical *(continued)*		
Physical illness	O	
Family history of mental illness (suicide)	H	
Childhood sexual/physical abuse	O	
Mental competency	M	
Interpersonal relations		
Work or school		L
Family		M
Spousal or partner	H	
Children	O	
Situational		
Living circumstances		M
Employment or school status		L
Financial status		L–M
Availability of guns	H	
Managed care setting	O	
Demographic		
Age	M	
Gender	H	
Marital status	L	
Race/ethnicity	O	
Overall risk ratings[b]	**High**	

FIGURE 1–2. Admission systematic suicide risk assessment: case example *(continued)*.

[a]Rate risk and protective factors present as low (L), moderate (M), high (H), nonfactor (O), or range (e.g., L–M, M–H).
[b]Judge overall suicide risk as low, moderate, high, or a range of risk.

Source. Adapted with permission from Simon 2004.

Assessment factors[a]	Risk	Protective
Individual		
Distinctive clinical features (prodrome)	O	
Religious beliefs		H
Reasons for living		M
Clinical		
Current attempt (lethality)	H	
Therapeutic alliance		M
Treatment adherence		H
Treatment benefit		M
Suicidal ideation (command hallucinations)	M	
Suicide intent	O	
Suicide plan	O	
Hopelessness	L	
Prior attempts (lethality)	L	
Panic attacks	O	
Psychic anxiety	O	
Loss of pleasure and interest	L	
Alcohol/drug abuse	M	
Depressive turmoil (mixed states)	O	
Diminished concentration	H	
Global insomnia	L	
Psychiatric diagnoses (Axis I and Axis II)	H	
Symptom severity	L–M	
Comorbidity	H	
Recent discharge from psychiatric hospital (within 3 months)	O	
Impulsivity/aggression	L	

FIGURE 1–3. Discharge systematic suicide risk assessment: case example.

Assessment factors[a]	Risk	Protective
Clinical *(continued)*		
Agitation (akathisia)	O	
Physical illness	H	
Family history of mental illness (suicide)	H	
Childhood sexual/physical abuse	O	
Mental competency	L	
Interpersonal relations		
Work or school		H
Family		H
Spousal or partner	L–M	
Children	O	
Situational		
Living circumstances		M
Employment or school status		H
Financial status		M
Availability of guns		O
Managed care setting	L–M	
Demographic		
Age	M	
Gender	L	
Marital status	L	
Race/ethnicity	O	
Overall risk ratings[b]	**Moderate**	

FIGURE 1–3. **Discharge systematic suicide risk assessment: case example *(continued)*.**

[a]Rate risk and protective factors present as low (L), moderate (M), high (H), nonfactor (O), or range (e.g., L–M, M–H).

[b]Judge overall suicide risk as low, moderate, high, or a range of risk.

Source. Adapted with permission from Simon 2004.

Malone et al. (2000) assessed inpatients with major depression for severity of depression, general psychopathology, suicide history, reasons for living, and hopelessness. The self-report Reasons for Living Inventory was used to measure beliefs that may act as preventive factors against suicide (Linehan et al. 1983). The total score for reasons for living was inversely correlated with the sum of scores for hopelessness, subjective depression, and suicidal ideation. The authors recommend including reasons for living in the clinical assessment and management of suicidal patients.

Protective factors against suicide may include family and social support, pregnancy, children at home, strong religious beliefs, and cultural sanctions against suicide (Institute of Medicine 2001). Some families, however, are not able to be supportive for a variety of reasons. Religious affiliation was associated with less suicidal behavior in depressed patients (Dervic et al. 2004). Severely depressed patients, however, may feel abandoned by God or may feel that God will understand, thus increasing their risk for suicide. Survival and coping skills, responsibility to family, and child-related concerns are protective factors (Linehan et al. 1983).

A therapeutic alliance between clinician and patient can be an important protective factor against suicide (Simon 1998). The therapeutic alliance is influenced by a number of factors, especially the nature and severity of the patient's illness. The extent to which the therapeutic alliance can influence a patient may change quickly from session to session. It cannot be assumed that a therapeutic alliance will be present and protective between sessions. Clinicians have been shocked and bewildered when a patient with whom the clinician felt a strong therapeutic alliance attempts or commits suicide between sessions. However, in a patient at risk for suicide, the absence of a therapeutic alliance should be considered a significant risk factor.

Protective factors, like risk factors, vary with the distinctive clinical presentation of the individual patient at suicide risk. An ebb and flow exists between suicide risk and protective factors. Protective factors are especially important for discharge planning. They are usually easier for patients to talk about than risk factors, thus tending to be overvalued by the patient or the clinician. Protective factors can be overcome by the acuteness and severity of mental illness (see Chapter 7, "Patients at Acute and Chronic High Risk for Suicide: Crisis Management").

Figure 1–1 divides assessment factors into five general categories: 1) individual, 2) clinical, 3) interpersonal, 4) situational, and 5) demo-

---

TABLE 1–2.   Sample suicide risk assessment note

- Suicide risk factors identified and weighed (low, moderate, high)
- Protective factors identified and weighed (low, moderate, high)
- Overall assessment rating (low, moderate, high, or range)
- Treatment and management intervention informed by the assessment
- Effectiveness of interventions evaluated

Source.   Adapted with permission from Simon 2004.

---

graphic. The practitioner ranks the risk and protective factors according to the patient's distinctive clinical presentation. Usually, acute, high-risk suicide risk factors are a focus of continuing clinical attention. "Acute" refers to the intensity (severity) and magnitude (duration) of symptoms, such as early morning awakening versus global insomnia. A high risk factor is supported by an evidence-based association with suicide (see Chapter 7, "Patients at Acute and Chronic High Risk for Suicide: Crisis Management").

A dimensional scale of low, moderate, high, or nonfactor reflecting the continuum of suicide risk is used. A final risk rating is a reasoned clinical judgment based on the overall assessment of the risk and protective factor pattern. The overall risk assessment informs treatment, safety management, and discharge decisions. The purpose of Figure 1–1 is to provide a *conceptual model* that encourages systematic suicide risk assessment. Assessments can be made in a time-efficient manner after thorough psychiatric examination and during continuing patient care. A concise, contemporaneous note that describes the clinician's suicide risk assessment and clinical decision-making process is adequate (see Table 1–2).

For instance, assessment factors can be rated as acute (the focus of clinical attention) or chronic (long-standing, usually static risk factors). After initial psychiatric examination and systematic suicide risk assessment, the clinician can evaluate the course of acute suicide risk factors that brought the patient to treatment. Modifiable and treatable suicide risk factors should be identified early and treated aggressively. For example, anxiety, depression, insomnia, and psychosis may respond rapidly to medications as well as to psychosocial interventions. Impulsivity may respond to treatment with anticonvulsants (Hollander et al. 2002) (Table 1–3). The clini-

TABLE 1–3. Modifiable and treatable suicide risk factors: some examples	
Depression	Impulsivity
Anxiety	Agitation
Panic attacks	Physical illness
Psychosis	Situation (e.g., family, work)
Sleep disorders	Lethal means (e.g., guns, drugs)
Substance abuse	Drug effects (e.g., akathisia)

Source.   Adapted with permission from Simon 2004.

cian should also identify, support, and, when possible, enhance protective factors. Psychosocial interventions can help mitigate or resolve interpersonal issues at home, work, or school. At discharge, a final systematic suicide risk assessment allows comparison with the initial office visit or hospital admission assessment to determine what is different.

Conclusion

Suicide risk assessment is a process, not an event. Suicide risk exists along a continuum that can vary from minute to minute, hour to hour, and day to day. Thus, assessments must be performed at several clinical junctures such as change of safety status, removal from seclusion and/or restraint, ward changes, prior to issuing passes, and at time of discharge. The suicide risk assessment process that follows the course of acute risk factors is illustrated in the case example presented earlier in the chapter. For outpatients, systematic suicide risk assessment is critical to clinical decision-making, especially regarding voluntary or involuntary hospitalization.

Patients with Axis I psychiatric disorders such as schizophrenia, anxiety disorders, major affective disorders, and substance use disorders often present with acute (state) suicide risk factors. Patients with Axis II disorders often display chronic (trait) suicide risk factors. Exacerbation of an Axis II disorder or comorbidity with an Axis I disorder (including substance abuse) may exacerbate and transform a chronic suicide risk factor, such as impulsivity, into an acute risk factor. A family history of mental illness, especially when associated with suicide, is an important chronic (static) risk factor. The offspring of mood-disordered patients who attempt suicide are at a markedly increased risk for suicide (Brent et al. 2002). In the Case Example, the patient's aunt was diagnosed as a "chronic schizophrenic," and a "manic-depressive" uncle had committed suicide. Comorbidity significantly increases the patient's risk for suicide (Kessler et al. 1999). Suicide risk increases with the total number of risk factors, providing a quasi-quantitative dimension to suicide risk factor assessment (Murphy et al. 1992).

Necessary (e.g., depression) and sufficient (e.g., situational) factors provide another assessment parameter. For example, the patient with major depression who also is experiencing a personal loss or work-related crisis presents with both necessary and sufficient suicide risk factors. Evaluating individual (e.g., distinctive or atypical suicide risk factors) and situational (e.g., loss) parameters can also be useful in suicide risk assessment. This parameter is a variant of the necessary and sufficient analysis.

Systematic suicide risk assessment encourages the gathering of relevant clinical information. Malone et al. (1995) found that on routine clinical assessments at admission, clinicians failed to document a history of suicidal behavior in 12 of 50 patients who were identified by research assessment as being depressed and as having attempted suicide. Fewer total suicide attempts were clinically reported than were shown by data of suicide attempts obtained by use of a comprehensive research assessment. Documentation of suicidal behavior was most accurate on hospital intake admission when a semi-structured format was used instead of discharge documentation by clinical assessment alone. Malone and colleagues suggested that use of semi-structured screening instruments may improve documentation and the detection of lifetime suicidal behavior.

Systematic suicide risk assessment of the patient's risk and protective factors is a gateway to improved information gathering that informs the identification, treatment, and management of patients at risk for suicide.

KEY CLINICAL CONCEPTS

- Fully commit time and effort to the ongoing assessment, treatment, and management of the patient at suicide risk.
- Conduct systematic suicide risk assessment to inform treatment and management of patients at risk for suicide.

- Identify treatable and modifiable suicide risk and protective factors early and treat aggressively. Delayed or ineffective treatment can result in a psychiatric condition becoming entrenched, causing patient demoralization, hopelessness, and adverse life consequences. Consider suicide reduction drugs such as lithium and clozapine in bipolar patients and schizophrenic patients, respectively.

- Do not use suicide prevention contracts in place of conducting systematic suicide risk assessments. Suicide risk assessment is a process, not an event.

- Contemporaneously document suicide risk assessments. Doing so facilitates good clinical care and is standard practice.

References

Addy CL: Statistical concepts of prediction, in Assessment and Prediction of Suicide. Edited by Maris RW, Berman AL, Maltsberger JT, et al. New York, Guilford, 1992, pp 218–232

American Psychiatric Association: Principles of Medical Ethics With Annotations Especially Applicable to Psychiatry. Washington, DC, American Psychiatric Association, 2001

American Psychiatric Association: Practice guideline for the assessment and treatment of patients with suicidal behaviors. Am J Psychiatry 160 (suppl 11):1–60, 2003

Baldessarini RJ: Lithium: effects on depression and suicide. J Clin Psychiatry 64:7, 2003

Baldessarini RJ, Pompili M, Tondo L: Bipolar disorder, in The American Psychiatric Publishing Textbook of Suicide Assessment and Management. Edited by Simon RI, Hales RE. Washington, DC, American Psychiatric Publishing, 2006, pp 277–299

Beck AT, Brown G, Berchick RJ, et al: Relationship between hopelessness and ultimate suicide: a replication with psychiatric outpatients. Am J Psychiatry 147:190–195, 1990

Beck AT, Steer RA, Ranieri WF: Scale for suicidal ideation: psychometric properties of a self-report version. J Clin Psychol 44:499–505, 1998

Black HC: Black's Law Dictionary, 7th Edition. St Paul, MN, West Publishing Group, 1999

Bongar B, Maris RW, Bertram AL, et al: Outpatient standards of care and the suicidal patient. Suicide Life Threat Behav 22:453–478, 1992

Brent DA: Assessment and treatment of the youthful suicidal patient. Ann N Y Acad Sci 932:106–131, 2001

Brent DA, Mann JJ: Family genetic studies, suicide and suicidal behavior. Am J Med Genet 133:13–24, 2005

Brent DA, Bridge J, Johnson BA, et al: Suicidal behavior runs in families. Arch Gen Psychiatry 53:1145–1152, 1996

Brent DA, Oquendo M, Birmaher B, et al: Familial pathways to early onset suicide attempt. Arch Gen Psychiatry 59:801–807, 2002

Breier A, Astrachan BM: Characterization of schizophrenic patients who commit suicide. Am J Psychiatry 141:206–209, 1984

Brodsky, BS, Malone KM, Ellis SP, et al: Characteristics of borderline personality disorder associated with suicidal behavior. Am J Psychiatry 154:1715–1719, 1997

Bronisch T: The typology of personality disorders–diagnostic problems and their relevance for suicidal behavior. Crisis 17:55–58, 1996

Busch KA, Clark DC, Fawcett J, et al: Clinical features of inpatient suicide. Psychiatr Ann 23:256–262, 1993

Busch KA, Fawcett J, Jacobs DG: Clinical correlates of inpatient suicide. J Clin Psychiatry 64:14–19, 2003

Clark DC, Fawcett J: An empirically based model of suicide risk assessment of patients with affective disorders, in Suicide and Clinical Practice. Edited by Jacobs DJ. Washington, DC, American Psychiatric Association, 1999, pp 55–73

Conwell Y, Duberstein PR: Suicide in elders. Ann N Y Acad Sci 932:132–150, 2001

Coryell W, Leon A, Winokur G, et al: Importance of psychotic features to long-term course in major depressive disorder. Am J Psychiatry 153:483–489, 1996

Dervic K, Oquendo MA, Grunebaum MF, et al: Religious affiliation and suicide attempt. Am J Psychiatry 161:2303–2308, 2004

Dube SR, Anda RF, Felitti VJ, et al: Childhood abuse, household dysfunction and the risk of attempted suicide throughout the lifespan: findings from the Adverse Childhood Experiences Study. JAMA 286:3089–3096, 2001

Duberstein P, Conwell Y: Personality disorders and completed suicide: a methodological and conceptual review. Clinical Psychology: Science and Practice 4:359–376, 1997

Evans J, Platts H, Liebenau A: Impulsiveness and deliberate self-harm: a comparison of "first-timers" and "repeaters." Acta Psychiatr Scand 93:378–380, 1996

Fawcett J: Treating impulsivity and anxiety in the suicidal patient. Ann N Y Acad Sci 932:94–105, 2001

Fawcett J, Scheftner WA, Clark DC, et al: Clinical predictors of suicide in patients with major affective disorders: a controlled prospective study. Am J Psychiatry 144:35–40, 1987

Fawcett J, Scheftner WA, Fogg L, et al: Time-related predictors of suicide in major affective disorder. Am J Psychiatry 147:1189–1194, 1990

Fawcett J, Clark DC, Busch KA: Assessing and treating the patient at suicide risk. Psychiatr Ann 23:244–255, 1993

Garno JL, Coldberg JF, Ramirez PM, et al: Bipolar disorder with comorbid cluster B personality features: impact on suicidality. J Clin Psychiatry 66:339–345, 2005

Gunderson JG, Ridolfi ME: Borderline personality disorder: suicide and self-mutilation. Ann N Y Acad Sci 932:61–77, 2002

Hall RC, Platt DE, Hall RC: Suicide risk assessment: a review of risk factors for suicide in 100 patients who made severe suicide attempts: evaluation of suicide risk in a time of managed care. Psychosomatics 40:18–27, 1999

Harkavy-Friedman JM, Kimhy D, Nelson EA., et al: Suicide attempts in schizophrenia: the role of command auditory hallucinations for suicide. J Clin Psychiatry 64:871–874, 2003

Harris CE, Barraclough B: Suicide as an outcome for mental disorders. Br J Psychiatry 170:205–228, 1997

Heikkinen ME, Henriksson MM, Erkki T, et al: Recent life events and suicide in personality disorders. J Nerv Ment Dis 185:373–381, 1997

Heila H, Isometsa ET, Henriksson MM, et al: Suicide and schizophrenia: a nationwide psychological autopsy study on age- and sex-specific clinical characteristics of 92 suicide victims with schizophrenia. Am J Psychiatry 154:1235–1242, 1997

Heila H, Heikkinen ME, Isometsa ET, et al: Life events and completed suicide in schizophrenia: a comparison of suicide victims with and without schizophrenia. Schizophr Bull 25:519–531, 1999

Hellerstein D, Frosch W, Koenigsbert HW: The clinical significance of command hallucinations. Am J Psychiatry 144:219–225, 1987

Heron M, Hoyert DL, Murphy SL, et al: Deaths: final data for 2006. National Vital Statistics Reports. April 2009. Available at: http://www.cdc.gov/nchs/data/nvsr/nvsr57/nvsr57_14.pdf. Accessed January 15, 2010.

Hollander E, Posner N, Cherkasky S: Neuropsychiatric aspects of aggression and impulse control disorders, in The American Psychiatric Press Textbook of Neuropsychiatry and Behavioral Neuroscience, 4th Edition. Edited by Yudofsky SC, Hales RE. Washington, DC, American Psychiatric Press, 2002, pp 579–596

Institute of Medicine: Reducing Suicide: A National Imperative. Washington, DC, National Academic Press, 2001, pp 2–4

Isometsa ET, Lonnqvist JK: Suicide attempts preceding completed suicide. Br J Psychiatry 173:531–535, 1998

Isometsa ET, Heikkinen ME, Martunen MJ, et al: The last appointment before suicide: is suicide intent communicated? Am J Psychiatry 152:919–922, 1995

Isometsa ET, Henriksson MM, Heikkinen ME, et al: Suicide among subjects with personality disorders. Am J Psychiatry 153:667–673, 1996

Jacobs DG, Brewer M, Klein-Benheim M: Suicide assessment: an overview and recommended protocol, in Guide to Suicide Assessment and Intervention. Edited by Jacobs DJ. San Francisco, CA, Jossey-Bass, 1999, pp 3–39

Juninger J: Predicting compliance with command hallucinations. Am J Psychiatry 147:245–247, 1990

Juninger J: Command hallucinations and the prediction of dangerousness. Psychiatr Serv 46:911–914, 1995

Kaplan M, Asnis GM, Lipschitz DS, et al: Suicidal behavior and abuse in psychiatric outpatients. Compr Psychiatry 36:229–235, 1995

Kasper ME, Rogers R, Adams PA: Dangerousness and command hallucinations: an investigation of psychotic inpatients. Bull Am Acad Psychiatry Law 24:219–224, 1996

Kessler RC, Borges G, Walters EE: Prevalence of and risk factors for lifetime suicide attempts in The National Comorbidity Survey. Arch Gen Psychiatry 55:617–626, 1999

Linehan MM: Cognitive Behavioral Treatment of Borderline Personality Disorder. New York, Guilford, 1993

Linehan MM, Goodstein JL, Nielsen SL, et al: Reasons for staying alive when you are thinking of killing yourself: the Reasons for Living Inventory. J Consult Clin Psychol 51:276–286, 1983

Linehan MM, Rizvi SL, Welch SS, et al: Psychiatric aspects of suicidal behaviour: personality disorders, in The International Handbook of Suicide and Attempted Suicide. Edited by Hawton K, van Heeringen K. New York, Wiley, 2000, pp 147–148

Loebel JP: Completed suicide in late life. Psychiatr Serv 56:260–262, 2005

Malone KM, Katalin S, Corbitt EM, et al: Clinical assessment versus research methods in the assessment of suicidal behavior. Am J Psychiatry 152:1601–1607, 1995

Malone KM, Oquendo MA, Hass GL, et al: Protective factors against suicidal acts in major depression: reasons for living. Am J Psychiatry 157:1084–1088, 2000

Mann JJ, Arango V: The neurobiology of suicidal behavior, in Guide to Suicide Assessment and Intervention. Edited by Jacobs D. San Francisco, CA, Jossey-Bass, 1999, pp 98–114

Mann JJ, Waternaux C, Haas GL, et al: Toward a clinical model of suicidal behavior in psychiatric patients. Am J Psychiatry 156:181–189, 1999

Mays D: Structured assessment methods may improve suicide prevention. Psychiatr Ann 34:367–372, 2004

McGirr A, Martin A, Ségun M, et al: Familial aggregation of suicide explained by cluster B traits: a three-group family study of suicide controlling for major depressive disorder. Am J Psychiatry 166:1124–1134, 2009

Meltzer HY: Treatment of suicidality in schizophrenia. Ann N Y Acad Sci 932:44–60, 2001

Meltzer HY, Okaly G: Reduction of suicidality during clozapine treatment of neuroleptic-resistant schizophrenia: impact of risk-benefit assessment. Am J Psychiatry 152:183–190, 1995

Meltzer HY, Alphs L, Green AI, et al: Clozapine treatment for suicidality in schizophrenia: international suicide prevention trial (InterSePT). Arch Gen Psychiatry 60:82–91, 2003a

Meltzer HY, Conley RR, de Leo D, et al: Intervention strategies for suicidality. Audiograph Series. J Clin Psychiatry 6:1–18, 2003b

Moeller FG, Barratt ES, Dougherty DM, et al: Psychiatric aspects of impulsivity. Am J Psychiatry 158:1783–1793, 2001

Monahan J, Steadman HJ: Violent storms and violent people: how meterology can inform risk communication in mental health law. Am J Psychol 51:931–938, 1996

Murphy GE, Wetzel RD, Robins E, et al: Multiple risk factors predict suicide in alcoholism. Arch Gen Psychiatry 49:459–462, 1992

O'Carroll PW, Berman AL, Maris RW, et al: Beyond the Tower of Babel: a nomenclature for suicidology. Suicide Life Threat Behav 26:237–252, 1996

Oquendo MA, Halberstam, Mann JJ: Risk factors for suicidal behavior: the utility and limitation of research instruments, in Standardized Evaluation in Clinical Practice. Edited by First MB. Washington, DC, American Psychiatric Publishing, 2003, pp 103–130

Perlis RH, Fraquas R, Fava M, et al: Prevalence and clinical correlates of irritability in major depressive disorder: a preliminary report from the Sequenced Treatment Alternatives to Relieve Depression study. J Clin Psychiatry 66:159–166, 2005

Peters PG: The quiet demise of deference to custom: malpractice law and the millennium. Wash Lee Law Rev 57:163, 2000

Pezawas L, Stamenkovic M, Reinhold J, et al: A longitudinal view of triggers and thresholds of suicidal behavior in depression. J Clin Psychiatry 63:866–873, 2002

Pokorny AD: Predictions of suicide in psychiatric patients: report of a prospective study. Arch Gen Psychiatry 40:249–257, 1983

Pokorny AD: Suicide prediction revisited. Suicide Life Threat Behav 23:1–10, 1993

Posternak MA, Zimmerman M: Is there a delay in the antidepressant effect? A meta-analysis. J Clin Psychiatry 66:148–158, 2005

Resnick PJ: Recognizing that the suicidal patient views you as an adversary. Curr Psychiatr 1:8, 2002

Robins E: The Final Months: Study of the Lives of 134 Persons Who Committed Suicide. New York, Oxford University Press, 1981

Roose SP, Glassman AH, Walsh BT, et al: Depression, delusions, and suicide. Am J Psychiatry 140:1159–1162, 1983

Roy A: Suicide in chronic schizophrenia. Br J Psychiatry 141:171–177, 1982

Roy A: Suicide. Baltimore, MD, Williams & Wilkins, 1986, pp 6, 93–94

Rudd MD, Joiner T, Rajab MH: Treating Suicidal Behavior: An Effective, Time-Limited Approach. New York, Guilford, 2001

Scheiber SC, Kramer TS, Adamowski SE: Core Competencies for Psychiatric Practice: What Clinicians Need to Know (A Report of the American Board of Psychiatry and Neurology). Washington, DC, American Psychiatric Publishing, 2003

Shaffer DA, Pfeffer CR, Bernet W, et al: Practice parameter for the assessment and treatment of children and adolescents with suicidal behavior. J Am Acad Child Adolesc Psychiatry 36 (suppl), 1997

Shea SC: The delicate art of eliciting suicidal ideation. Psychiatr Ann 34:385–400, 2004

Simon RI: Clinical Psychiatry and the Law, 2nd Edition. Washington, DC, American Psychiatric Press, 1992

Simon RI: The suicidal patient, in The Mental Health Practitioner and the Law: A Comprehensive Handbook. Edited by Lifson LE, Simon RI. Cambridge, MA, Harvard University Press, 1998, pp 329–343

Simon RI: Psychiatry and Law for Clinicians, 3rd Edition. Washington, DC, American Psychiatric Publishing, 2001, p 147

Simon RI: Suicide risk assessment: what is the standard of care? J Am Acad Psychiatry Law 30:340–344, 2002

Simon RI: Assessing and Managing Suicide Risk: Guidelines for Clinically Based Risk Management. Washington, DC, American Psychiatric Publishing, 2004

Simon RI: Standard of care testimony: best practice or reasonable care? J Am Acad Psychiatry Law 33:8–11, 2005

Simon RI: Suicide risk assessment forms: form over substance? J Am Acad Psychiatry Law 37:290–293, 2009

Simon RI, Gutheil TG: Clinician factors associated with increased risk for patient suicide. Psychiatr Ann 330:1–4, 2004

Simon RI, Shuman DW: Clinical Manual of Psychiatry and Law. Washington, DC, American Psychiatric Publishing, 2007

Simon TR, Swann AC, Powell KE, et al: Characteristics of impulsive suicide attempts and attempters. Suicide Life Threat Behav 32(suppl):49–59, 2001

Stanford EJ, Goetz RR, Bloom JD: The no harm contract in the emergency assessment of suicide risk. J Clin Psychiatry 55:344–348, 1994

Stepakoff v Kantar, 473 N.E.2d 1131, 1134 (Mass 1985)

Stone M: Natural history of borderline patients treated by intensive hospitalization. Br J Psychiatry 10:185–206, 1987

Stone M: Long-term outcome in personality disorders. Br J Psychiatry 162:299–313, 1993

Suominen KH, Isometsa ET, Henriksson MM, et al: Suicide attempts and personality disorder. Acta Psychiatr Scand 102:118–125, 2000

Taylor CB (ed): How to Practice Evidence-Based Psychiatry: Basic Principles. Washington, DC, American Psychiatric Publishing, 2010

Vythilingam M, Chen J, Bremmer JD, et al: Psychotic depression and mortality. Am J Psychiatry 160:574–576, 2003

Warman DM, Forman E, Henriques GR, et al: Suicidality and psychosis: beyond depression and hopelessness. Suicide Life Threat Behav 34:77–86, 2004

Weisman AD, Worden JW: Risk-rescue rating in suicide assessment. Arch Gen Psychiatry 26:553–560, 1972

Zimmerman M, Chelminski I: Generalized anxiety disorder in patients with major depression: is DSM-IV's hierarchy correct? Am J Psychiatry 160:504–512, 2003

Zimmerman M, Chelminski I, McDermut W: Major depressive disorder and Axis I diagnostic comorbidity. J Clin Psychiatry 63:187–193, 2002

CHAPTER 2

Enhancing Suicide Risk Assessment Through Evidence-Based Psychiatry

SUICIDE risk assessment is a core competency that psychiatrists are expected to acquire (Scheiber et al. 2003). The purpose of suicide risk assessment is to identify treatable and modifiable risk and protective factors that inform the patient's treatment and safety management. Evidence-based psychiatry can enhance suicide risk assessment by diminishing reliance on lore, tradition, and unaided clinical impression. Acceptance of expert opinion solely based on respect for authority is giving way to evidence-based medicine.

Patients at risk for suicide often confront the psychiatrist with life-threatening emergencies. Most clinicians rely on the clinical interview and

Adapted from "Suicide Risk Assessment: Evidence-Based Psychiatry." Guttmacher Award Lecture. Presented at the 158th Annual Meeting of the American Psychiatric Association. Atlanta, GA, May 21, 2005.

certain valued questions and observations to assess suicide risk (Sullivan and Bongar 2006). The psychiatrist, unlike the general physician, does not have laboratory tests and sophisticated diagnostic instruments available to assess the suicidal patient. For example, in evaluating an emergency cardiac patient, the clinician can order a number of diagnostic tests and procedures such as electrocardiogram, serial enzymes, imaging, and catheterization. The psychiatrist's diagnostic instrument is systematic suicide risk assessment that is informed by evidence-based psychiatry.

No suicide risk assessment *method* has been empirically tested for reliability and validity (Simon 2006a). The standard of care encompasses a range of reasoned approaches to suicide risk assessment.

Utilizing evidence-based psychiatry is best practice. It is not, however, a standard-of-care requirement. Moreover, the law does not require the mental health professional to provide ideal, best-practice, or even good patient care; the clinician's legal duty is to provide adequate patient care.

Sackett et al. (1996) define evidence-based medicine as "The conscientious, explicit, and judicious use of current best evidence in making decisions about the care of individual patients" (pp. 71–72). The method of evidence-based psychiatry is described in a volume edited by Taylor (2010). The preferred study designs for determining harm (risk) are cohort and case-control studies. Online evidence-based psychiatric information sources include National Electronic Library for Mental Health (comprehensive sources), Evidence-Based Mental Health (structured abstracts), Cochrane Database of Systematic Reviews (systematic reviews), PubMed (original articles), and PsycINFO (comprehensive sources).

Evidence-Based Suicide Risk and Protective Factors: Some Examples

In Table 2–1, examples of evidence-based suicide risk factors are arranged according to the hierarchy of supporting evidence. The hierarchy of evidence for studies of harm (risk) includes systematic reviews (meta-analysis), the highest level of evidence, followed by cohort studies (prospective or retrospective) and case-control studies (retrospective) (Taylor 2010). In a retrospective cohort study, a historical cohort is identified through existing records for outcomes of interest at initiation of the study. Dependence on existing records, however, raises questions

---

TABLE 2–1. Suicide risk and protective factors: examples of evidence-based studies

---

Suicide risk factors

Systematic reviews (meta-analysis)

  Psychiatric diagnosis (Harris et al. 1997; Kessler et al. 1999)

  Physical illness (Harris et al. 1994; Quan et al. 2002)

Cohort studies

  Deliberate self-harm (Cooper et al. 2005)

  Anxiety (Fawcett et al. 1990)

  Child abuse (Brown et al. 1999; Dube et al. 2005)

Case-control studies

  Violent threats: impulsivity and aggression (Conner et al. 2001; Dumais et al. 2005; Mann et al. 2008)

  Melancholia (Grunebaum et al. 2004)

  Comorbidity (Beautrais et al. 1996; Hawton and Zahl 2003)

Suicide protective factors

Case-control studies

  Protective factors (Malone et al. 2000)

  Religious affiliation (Dervic et al. 2004)

  Reasons for living (Reason for Living Inventory) (Linehan et al. 1983)

---

of data quality (Taylor 2010). Non-evidence-based suicide risk factors are based on case reports, case series, and, lastly, clinical opinion and clinical consensus. Clinical opinion and consensus are important in suicide risk assessment if buttressed by evidence-based studies. The extensive suicide literature contains many well-designed studies regarding suicide risk factors that are beyond the scope of this chapter.

Systematic Reviews (Meta-Analysis)

Psychiatric Diagnosis

Harris and Barraclough (1997), in a systematic review (i.e., meta-analysis), abstracted 249 reports from the medical literature regarding the mortality of mental disorders. They compared the number of suicides in individuals with mental disorders with the number of those expected in the general population. The standardized mortality ratio (SMR) is a measure of the relative risk of suicide for a particular disorder compared with the expected rate in the general population (SMR of 1). The SMR was calculated for each disorder by dividing observed mortality by expected mortality (see Chapter 5, "Psychiatric Disorders and Suicide Risk"; Table 5–1).

The highest relative risk for suicide was associated with eating disorders. The SMR for eating disorders was significantly higher than the SMRs for major affective disorders and substance abuse. All psychiatric disorders except mental retardation *were* associated with an increased risk of suicide. Making an accurate psychiatric diagnosis—one of the most important indicators of risk for suicide—is essential to competent suicide risk assessment (Simon 2004).

Physical Illness

Physical illness, especially in the elderly, is associated with suicide risk. Quan et al. (2002), in a systematic review, found that the psychiatrically ill elderly with any of the following illnesses were more likely to complete suicide than those without the illness: cancer, prostatic disorder (excluding prostatic cancer), and chronic pulmonary disease.

In a statistical overview, Harris and Barraclough (1994) identified a number of specific medical illnesses that were associated with increased suicide risk: HIV/AIDS, malignant neoplasms as a group, head and neck cancers, Huntington's chorea, multiple sclerosis, peptic ulcer, renal disease, spinal cord injury, and systemic lupus erythematosus. Recognition of specific medical conditions that are associated with increased risk of suicide aids the clinician's suicide risk assessment.

Evidence-Based Studies

Cohort Studies

Deliberate self-harm. In a prospective cohort study of 7,968 deliberate self-harm patients, Cooper et al. (2005) found an approximately 30-fold increase in risk of suicide compared with the general population during a 4-year follow-up period. Suicide rates were highest within the first 6 months after the initial self-harm. The authors underscored the importance of early intervention following self-harm. Female patients were at high risk for suicide.

Hawton and Zahl (2003) conducted a follow-up study of 11,583 deliberate self-harm patients who presented to a hospital between 1978 and 1997. The authors found a significant and persistent risk of suicide. In this study, the risk was far higher in men than in women. In both men and women, suicide increased markedly with age at initial presentation.

Anxiety.   Fawcett et al. (1990) identified short-term suicide risk factors, derived from a 10-year prospective study of 954 patients with major affective disorders that were statistically significant for suicide within 1 year of assessment. The risk factors included panic attacks, psychic anxiety, loss of pleasure and interest, moderate alcohol abuse, diminished concentration, global insomnia, and depressive turmoil (agitation). Clinical interventions directed at treating the anxiety-related symptoms in patients with major affective disorders can rapidly diminish suicide risk (Fawcett 2001).

Child abuse.   An essential part of the psychiatric examination and systematic risk assessment is inquiry about childhood abuse as a risk factor for suicide. Dube et al. (2005) conducted a retrospective cohort study of 17,337 adult HMO members from 1995 to 1997. Compared with individuals who reported no sexual abuse, men and women who experienced childhood sexual abuse were more than twice as likely to have a history of suicide attempts. In patients with suicidal behaviors, the clinician should ask about sexual abuse (Bebbington et al. 2009).

Brown et al. (1999) studied a cohort of 776 randomly selected children from age 5 years to adulthood over a 17-year period. Adolescents and young adults with a history of childhood abuse were three times more likely to become depressed or suicidal than individuals without such a history. Childhood sexual abuse effects were the largest and most independent of associated factors. The risk of repeated suicide attempts was eight times greater when there was a history of sexual abuse.

The nature and extent of childhood sexual abuse is associated with the severity of suicide risk. Fergusson et al. (1996) followed a birth cohort of 1,019 males and females from birth to age 18 years. There was a consistent relationship between the extent of child sexual abuse and risk of a psychiatric disorder. Individuals reporting there had been sexual intercourse were at highest risk for psychiatric disorders and suicidal behaviors.

Case-Control Studies

Violent threats: impulsivity and aggression. Violent threats or behavior toward others is a suicide risk factor. Clinicians more commonly encounter patients who threaten violence against themselves. Violence, however, has a vector; it can be directed at oneself, at others, or both, as in murder-suicide. Impulsive aggression is the response to frustration or provocation with hostility and aggression.

Conner et al. (2001), in a case-control study, found that violent behavior in the last year of life was a significant risk factor for suicide. The relationship was especially strong in individuals with no history of alcohol abuse, in younger individuals, and in women. In the study, 753 suicide victims were compared with 2,115 accident victims. Violent behavior distinguished suicide victims from accident victims. The findings were not attributable to alcohol use disorders alone.

Dumais et al. (2005), using a case-control design, indicated that higher levels of impulsivity and aggression were associated with suicide. In the study, 104 male suicide completers who died during an episode of major depression were compared with 74 living depressed male subjects. Current (6-month prevalence) alcohol abuse/dependence and current drug abuse/dependence disorders increased the risk of suicide in individuals with major depression. Impulsive-aggressive personality disorders and alcohol/substance abuse were independent predictors of suicide in individuals with major depression.

In a retrospective study of 408 patients with mood, schizophrenia spectrum, or personality disorders who externally directed aggression, Mann et al. (2008) distinguished past suicide attempters from nonattempters. The risk of future suicide attempts also increased in the aggression group. McGirr et al. (2009) showed that the association of impulsive-aggressive and Cluster B personality traits was a marker for early-onset suicidal behaviors.

Melancholia. Do melancholic features associated with major depressive disorder confer a higher risk of suicide attempts than in nonmelancholic major depression? Grunebaum et al. (2004), in a case-control study, compared suicide attempts in 377 melancholic with nonmelancholic patients. Melancholia was associated with more serious past suicide attempts and increased probability of suicide attempts during follow up. Although major depression is associated with a high risk of suicide, melancholia is a less commonly recognized feature of major depression that may further increase the risk of suicide attempts or completions (see Chapter 5, "Psychiatric Disorders and Suicide Risk").

Comorbidity. Psychiatric patients often present with more than one psychiatric disorder. For example, a bipolar patient may be diagnosed with borderline personality disorder and substance abuse. Beautrais et al. (1996) found that individuals who made serious suicide attempts had high rates of comorbid mental disorders. In the study, 302 consecutive individuals who made serious suicide attempts were compared with 1,028 randomly selected subjects. The risk of suicide increased with increasing comorbidity—subjects with two or more disorders were at 89.7 times increased risk for suicide than those with no psychiatric disorder. Comorbidity is an independent suicide risk factor.

Employing a case-control design, Hawton and Zahl (2003) assessed 111 patients who attempted suicide (72 female and 39 male). They found that more patients with comorbid disorders had made previous suicide attempts and repeated attempts during the follow-up period. Comorbidity of Axis I disorders and personality disorders was present in 44% of patients.

In a national population survey of 5,877 respondents between 1990 and 1992, Kessler et al. (1999) discovered that a dose-response relationship existed between the number of comorbid psychiatric disorders and suicide attempts.

Protective Factors: Reasons for Living

Malone et al. (2000) assessed 84 patients with a DSM-III-R diagnosis of major depression. Of the 84 patients, 45 had attempted suicide and 39 had not. The depressed patients who had not attempted suicide expressed more responsibility toward family, more fear of social disapproval, more moral objections to suicide, greater coping and survival skills, and more fear of suicide than depressed patients who had attempted suicide. The authors concluded that the assessment of reasons for living should be part of the assessment of patients at risk for suicide.

The Linehan Reasons for Living Inventory (Linehan et al. 1983) assesses the strength of a patient's commitment not to die. The inventory is a 48-item self-report measure that takes about 10 minutes to administer. A 72-item version is also available. Internal consistency is high. The inventory's test-retest reliability is moderately high for 3 weeks. The inventory is sensitive to improvements in depression and hopelessness and in suicidal patients with borderline personality disorder who are receiving treatment.

How important are religious beliefs for preventing suicide? Dervic et al. (2004) assessed 371 depressed inpatients for religious affiliation. Patients without a religious affiliation had significantly more suicide attempts and more first-degree relatives who had completed suicide than patients with religious affiliations. Unaffiliated patients were younger and less often married, and fewer had children. They also had less contact with family members. Patients with no religious affiliation had fewer reasons for living, especially in the category of moral objections to suicide. There was no difference in subjective and objective depression, hopelessness, or stressful life events. The authors concluded that greater moral objection to suicide and lower aggression level in terms of self-harm in religiously affiliated patients may act as protective factors against suicide attempts.

However, religious beliefs may not necessarily be a protective factor against suicide. In some patients, religious beliefs can be challenged by severe mental illness. For example, a bipolar patient stated hopelessly that "God has forsaken me." A devout, severely depressed patient hurled "blasphemous" insults at God. In a twist, religion became a facilitating risk factor in a case in which a suicidal patient stated, "God will forgive me if I kill myself." Severe mental illness can overcome a patient's protective factors.

Clinical Experience and Consensus

Case reports, case series, and clinical consensus, though not evidence-based, can aid suicide risk assessment. For example, in a systematic review of the relevant literature, Hansen (2001) found that akathisia could not be definitively linked to suicidal behavior. In individual cases, however, clinical judgment may determine that akathisia adds to the patient's total illness burden, thus potentially increasing suicide risk. Evidence-based studies must be interpreted through the lens of the clinician's education, training, experience, and reasoned clinical judgment.

Lore, tradition, myths, caprice, anxiety, defensiveness, and preconceptions are some factors that can lead to uncritical acceptance and perpetuation of substandard, pseudo-suicide assessments. Mental health professionals must do more than merely ask patients if they are suicidal and then record, "No SI, HI, or CFS" (no suicidal ideation, homicidal ideation, or contracts for safety). Suicide risk assessment necessitates identifying multiple risk and protective factors that guide treatment and management.

The so-called suicide prevention contract (SPC), also referred to as a "no-harm" contract, is a classic example of misconception. The SPC often masquerades as a protective factor, but it can be an iatrogenic suicide risk factor. For example, the SPC can falsely reassure the clinician, preempting adequate suicide risk assessments, and increasing the patient's risk for suicide (Simon 2004). No studies demonstrate that the SPC is effective in preventing suicide attempts or completions (Stanford et al. 1994). Clinician anxiety is unavoidable in the treatment of suicidal patients; it is a reality of clinical practice. Evidence-based suicide risk assessments can help increase the clinician's comfort in treating and managing suicidal patients.

Managed care settings can become a potential suicide risk factor, if clinicians permit third-party payers to dictate short length of stays that result in the premature discharge of suicidal patients. Safety contracts are often relied on with severely mentally ill suicidal patients who are rapidly treated and discharged, which compounds suicide risk.

Beyond evidence-based general suicide risk factors, patients at high risk for suicide have individual, "signature" symptoms and behaviors that are associated with suicide risk. Signature risk factors recur during subsequent suicide crises. A patient's distinctive suicide risk factor patterns should receive high priority in the identification and assessment of suicide risk. For example, a guarded, schizophrenic patient with a severe stutter would speak clearly when at high risk for suicide. Once his stutter returned, he was discharged from the hospital at low suicide risk. This individual, specific behavior was repeated a number of times. It was considered by the clinician to be a reliable behavioral indicator of suicide risk. The assessment of behavioral risk factors is important, especially with guarded or deceptive suicidal patients (see Chapter 4: "Behavioral Risk Assessment of the Guarded Suicidal Patient"). Employing evidence-based risk factors in suicide assessment is important, but knowing a patient's unique suicide risk profile is critical.

Conclusion

Suicide risk assessment is a core competency that psychiatrists are expected to possess. The purpose of suicide risk assessment is to identify treatable and modifiable risk and protective factors that inform the patient's treatment and safety management requirements. Unaided clinical experience can lead to impressionistic, substandard suicide risk assessments. The psychiatrist's diagnostic instrument is systematic suicide risk assessment that is informed by evidence-based psychiatry.

Clinician anxiety is unavoidable in the treatment of suicidal patients. Evidence-based suicide risk assessments can help increase clinicians' confidence in their assessments. Ultimately, evidence-based studies must be interpreted through the psychiatrist's reasoned clinical judgment.

KEY CLINICAL CONCEPTS

- Suicide risk assessment is informed by evidence-based psychiatry.

- Unaided clinical experience can lead to impressionistic, substandard suicide risk assessments.

- Evidence-based suicide risk assessments can help increase clinicians' confidence in their assessments.

- The preferred study designs for determining risk are cohort and case-control studies.

- Evidence-based psychiatry enhances suicide risk assessment by dispelling reliance on lore and tradition.

References

Beautrais L, Joyce PR, Mulder RT, et al: Prevalence and comorbidity of mental disorders in persons making serious suicide attempts: a case control study. Am J Psychiatry 153:1009–1014, 1996

Bebbington PE, Cooper C, Minot S, et al: Suicide attempts, gender and sexual abuse; data from the 2000 British Psychiatric Morbidity Survey. Am J Psychiatry 166:1135–1140, 2009

Brown J, Cohen P, Johnson JG, et al: Childhood abuse and neglect: specificity of effects on adolescent and young adult depression and suicidality. J Am Acad Child Adolesc Psychiatry 38:1490–1496, 1999

Conner KR, Cox C, Duberstein PR, et al: Violence, alcohol, and completed suicide: a case control study. Am J Psychiatry 158:1701–1705, 2001

Cooper J, Kapur N, Webb R, et al: Suicide after deliberate self-harm: a 4-year cohort study. Am J Psychiatry 162:297–303, 2005

Dervic K, Uquendo MA, Grunebaum MF, et al: Religious affiliation and suicide attempt. Am J Psychiatry 161:2303–2308, 2004

Dube SR, Anda RF, Whitfield CL, et al: Long–term consequences of childhood sexual abuse by gender of victim. Am J Prev Med 28:430–438, 2005

Dumais A, Lesage AD, Alda M, et al: Risk factors for suicide completion in major depression: a case control study of impulsive and aggressive behaviors in men. Am J Psychiatry 162:2116–2124, 2005

Fawcett J: Treating impulsivity and anxiety in the suicidal patient. Ann N Y Acad Sci 932:94–105, 2001

Fawcett J, Scheftner WA, Fogg L, et al: Time related predictors of suicide in major affective disorders: a controlled study. Am J Psychiatry 147:1189–1194, 1990

Fergusson DM, Horwood LJ, Lynsky MT: Childhood sexual abuse and psychiatric disorder in young adulthood: psychiatric outcomes of childhood sexual abuse. J Am Acad Child Adolesc Psychiatry 35:1365–1374, 1996

Grunebaum MF, Galfalvy HC, Oquendo MA, et al: Melancholia and the probability and lethality of suicide attempts. Br J Psychiatry 184:534–535, 2004

Hansen L: A critical review of akathisia and its possible association with suicidal behavior. Hum Psychopharmacol 116:495–505, 2001

Harris EC, Barraclough BM: Suicide as an outcome for medical disorders. Medicine (Baltimore) 73:281–296, 1994

Harris CE, Barraclough B: Suicide as an outcome for mental disorders. Br J Psychiatry 170:205–228, 1997

Hawton K, Zahl DA: Suicide following deliberate self-harm: long-term follow-up of patients who presented to a general hospital. Br J Psychiatry 182:537–542, 2003

Kessler RC, Borges G, Walters EE: Prevalence of and risk factors for lifetime suicide attempts in the National Comorbidity Study. Arch Gen Psychiatry 56:617–626, 1999

Linehan MM, Goodstein JL, Nielsen SL, et al: Reasons for staying alive when you are thinking of killing yourself: The Reasons for Living Inventory. J Consult Clin Psychol 51:276–286, 1983

Malone KM, Oquendo MA, Hass GL, et al: Protective factors against suicidal acts in major depression: reasons for living. Am J Psychiatry 157:1084–1088, 2000

Mann JJ, Ellis SP, Waternaux CM, et al: Classification trees distinguish suicide attempters in major psychiatric disorders: a model of clinical decision making. J Clin Psychiatry 69:23–31, 2008

McGirr A, Alda M, Séquin M, et al: Familial aggregation of suicide explained by Cluster B traits: a three group family study of suicide controlling for major depressive disorder. Am J Psychiatry 166:1124–1134, 2009

Quan H, Arboleda-Florez J, Fick GH, et al: Association between physical illness and suicide among the elderly. Soc Psychiatry Psychiatr Epidemiol 37:190–197, 2002

Sackett DE, Rosenberg WMC, Gray JA, et al: Evidence-based medicine: what it is and what it isn't. BMJ 312:71–72, 1996

Scheiber SC, Kramer TA, Adamowski SE: Core Competence for Psychiatric Practice: What Clinicians Need to Know (A Report of the American Board of Psychiatry and Neurology). Washington, DC, American Psychiatric Publishing, 2003

Simon RI: Assessing and Managing Suicide Risk: Guidelines for Clinically Based Risk Management. Washington, DC, American Psychiatric Publishing, 2004

Simon RI: Clinically based risk management of the suicidal patient: avoiding malpractice litigation, in The American Psychiatric Publishing Textbook of Suicide Assessment and Management. Edited by Simon RI, Hales RE. Washington, DC, American Psychiatric Publishing, 2006a, pp 545–575

Simon RI: Suicide risk assessment: assessing the unpredictable, in The American Psychiatric Publishing Textbook of Suicide Assessment and Management. Edited by Simon RI, Hales RE. Washington, DC, American Psychiatric Publishing, 2006b, pp 1–32

Simon RI: Behavioral risk assessment of the guarded suicidal patient. Suicide Life Threat Behav 38:517–522, 2008

Stanford EJ, Goetz RR, Bloom JD: The no harm contract in the emergency assessment of suicide risk. J Clin Psychiatry 55:344–348, 1994

Sullivan GR, Bongar B: Psychological testing in suicide risk management in avoiding malpractice litigation, in The American Psychiatric Publishing Textbook of Suicide Assessment and Management. Edited by Simon RI, Hales RE. Washington, DC, American Psychiatric Publishing, 2006, pp 177–196

Taylor CB (ed): How to Practice Evidence-Based Psychiatry: Basic Principles. Washington, DC, American Psychiatric Publishing, 2010

CHAPTER 3

Assessing and Enhancing Protective Factors Against Suicide Risk

SUICIDE risk assessment identifies counterbalancing modifiable and treatable risk and protective factors that inform the clinician's treatment and safety management of the patient at risk for suicide. Although the suicide literature frequently refers to protective factors, much less is written about the systematic assessment of protective factors that support the suicidal patient's life instincts (Lizardi et al. 2007). Protective factors require the same thorough assessment as risk factors. An assessment in which only risk factors are considered is incomplete. It does not inform the clinician regarding the patient's *overall* suicide risk. Thus, suicide risk may be erroneously assessed as too high, causing the clinician to be unduly defensive and restrictive in the patient's management. As a result, the opportunity to identify and mobilize protective factors is compromised.

A search of Google Scholar, PubMed, Medline, Cochrane Library, Ovid, and the National Electronic Library for Mental Health using the search term "suicidal patient protective factors" yielded relevant evidence-based studies regarding protective factors against suicide risk.

The studies discussed ahead focus on internal and external protective factor domains. However, both internal and external protective factors often coexist. *Internal protective factors* reflect the patient's characterological and psychological strengths (e.g., coping skills). *External protective factors* identify the patient's current life circumstances and relationships (e.g., family support). Internal protective factors often improve with treatment but usually take time. External protective factors are often amenable to current management. Protective factors vary with age, gender, race/ethnicity, culture, and other demographic factors.

Linehan et al. (1983) developed the Reasons for Living Inventory (RFLI), a self-report instrument that identifies protective factors against suicide. The RFLI consists of six subscales: 1) survival and coping beliefs, 2) responsibility to family, 3) child-related concerns, 4) fear of suicide, 5) fear of social disapproval, and 6) moral objections to suicide. Reliability and validity for the RFLI have been established. Survival and coping beliefs, responsibility to family, and child-related concerns were most useful in differentiating between suicidal and nonsuicidal groups.

Malone et al. (2000) assessed 84 inpatients with major depression. Of these, 45 had attempted suicide. The depressed patients were administered the RFLI. Depressed patients who had not attempted suicide (n=39) expressed more sense of responsibility toward family, more fear of social disapproval, more moral objections to suicide, greater survival and coping skills, and greater fear of suicide than did depressed patients who attempted suicide. The authors concluded that the evaluation of reasons for living should be part of the suicide assessment of patients.

Dervic et al. (2004) assessed 371 depressed inpatients according to religious or nonreligious affiliation. Unaffiliated patients made significantly more suicide attempts, had more first-degree relative suicides, were younger, were less frequently married, less often had children, and had fewer contact with family members.

Oquendo et al. (2005) addressed protective factors as a function of culture. Patients (N=460) with major depression, bipolar disorder, and schizophrenia were evaluated regarding depression and lifetime suicidal behaviors. On the RFLI, Latinos scored higher than non-Latinos on the survival and coping beliefs, responsibility to family, and moral objections to suicide. The authors posited that Latinos may espouse cultural values that protect against suicidal behavior.

Borowsky et al. (2001) reviewed data from the National Longitudinal Study of Adolescent Health, conducted in 1995 and 1996. A nationally representative sample of 13,110 students from grades 7 through 12 were interviewed 11 months apart. Protective factors against suicide attempts were determined in African American, Hispanic, and white girls and boys. Perceived family connectedness was significantly protective for all youth. For girls, emotional well-being was also protective for all racial/ethnic groups. Grade point average was an additional protective factor for all boys. High parental expectations for school achievement, more people living at home, and religious beliefs were protective for some of the boys. Available counseling services at school and parental presence at key times during the day were protective for some girls, but not for boys.

Shenassa et al. (2004) used data from the 1993 National Mortality Followback Survey sample of 22,957 deaths, representing 2,215,000 people, to analyze the protective effect of safer firearm storage practices. Individuals who stored their firearms locked or unloaded or both were less likely to complete suicide by firearms. The study demonstrated that the strongest protective effect of such practices occurred among suicide victims who engaged in impulsive suicidal behaviors.

In a case-control study of adolescent suicides and accessibility to firearms at home, Brent et al. (1991) compared 47 suicide victims from a consecutive case sample with two inpatient control groups, 47 patients who had attempted suicide, and 47 who had never been suicidal. Method of storing firearms did not differ in suicide association among the three groups, so that even guns that were locked or separated from ammunition were associated with firearm suicides. Guns were twice as likely to be found in the homes of adolescents who completed suicide as in the homes of suicide attempters. The availability of guns in the home, independent of storage method, increased the suicide risk among adolescents. Removing guns from the home reduces the risk of suicide and enhances the patient's protective environment (for detailed discussion, see Chapter 9, "Gun Safety Management of Suicidal Patients: A Collaborative Approach").

Marzuk et al. (1997) determined the risk of suicide during pregnancy by analyzing autopsy reports of all female residents of New York

City, ages 10–44 years, who completed suicide between 1990 and 1993. The race-adjusted standardized mortality ratio for suicide was 0.33, only one-third of the expected rate. The authors concluded that despite the mood swings and stresses of pregnancy and childbirth, pregnant women have a significantly lower risk of suicide than women of childbearing age who are not pregnant.

Fawcett et al. (1987), in a prospective study of 954 patients with major affective disorders, found an association between persons completing suicide and persons not living with a child under age 18 years. Thus, living with a child who is under 18 years old acts as a protective factor against suicide if the patient does not have a psychotic depression (Fawcett 2006). Much depends, however, on the parent-child relationship and the mental health of the child.

General and Individual Protective Factors

No protective factor is absolute. The acuteness and severity of mental illness can nullify protective factors. Moreover, evidence-based studies identify general protective factors that may not apply to individual patients. For example, Dervic et al. (2004) found religious affiliation to be a protective factor against suicide. However, the devout, severely depressed patient may feel abandoned by God or feel that God will understand and forgive suicide. The fact that a protective factor is evidence-based does not ensure its applicability to a specific patient. Evidence-based protective factors cannot be applied in a stock fashion.

The protective factors identified by the RFLI in the Linehan et al. (1983) study and replicated by Malone et al. (2000) represent internal core character and personality traits that perfectionist, high-functioning, successful individuals often possess. When such individuals become depressed, they often despair over the loss of highly valued coping and survival skills; they feel hopeless and are at high risk for suicide.

As part of a systematic suicide risk assessment, the RFLI can assist the clinician in determining the severity of the patient's depression and the patient's response to treatment. Protective factors such as survival and coping skills, despite being enduring traits, may be temporarily disabled by severe depression or other psychiatric disorders and medication side effects. Electroconvulsive therapy (ECT) can produce transient confusion, disorientation, and memory deficits.

Patients may emphasize protective factors while minimizing risk factors for a variety of reasons (e.g., to maintain denial or to obtain an early discharge from the hospital). Protective factors are easier for patients to talk about, thus tending to be overvalued by the patient and the clinician. In addition, the clinician may assume that the patient wants to get well and is cooperative (Resnick 2002).

General protective factors require further scrutiny. Protective factors are varied, often in ways that the clinician can only learn from evaluating the individual patient (e.g., pets, pictures of loved ones). Protective factors cannot be accepted at face value. An assumed protective factor, on further examination, may be a stealth suicide risk factor (e.g., suicide prevention contract). In another example, family support may be insufficient or actually destructive. Some families or family members are sicker than the patient. "Family connectedness" (Borowsky et al. 2001) is a general protective factor, but it lacks specificity and meaning unless it is further evaluated. Having a child at home who is under 18-years-old is an evidence-based general protective factor (Fawcett 2006; Veevers 1973). However, having an impulsive, acting-out, drug-abusing adolescent under age 18 years can also be a significant risk factor for suicide.

Clinical lore holds that pregnant women rarely complete suicide. Pregnancy, however, may not be a welcomed event for some women. Also, women with prior or current mental illnesses who become pregnant are often at increased risk for depression and suicide. Pregnancy is not an absolute protective factor. The Marzuk et al. (1997) study mentioned previously showed that pregnant women still completed suicide, though at one-third the expected rate.

Restoring and Enhancing Protective Factors

Restoring and enhancing internal protective factors (e.g., character, personality, psychological defenses) occur as consequences of effective treatment of the patient's psychiatric disorder. Inpatient discharge and follow-up planning are informed by the current status of protective factors. In the outpatient treatment of the patient at risk for suicide, an opportunity usually exists to improve internal coping and survival skills. Depending on the type of treatment, external protective factors may not be engaged directly (e.g., involving family). Enhancement of external protective factors is a treatment and management issue.

In the inpatient setting, external protective factors (e.g., relationships, life situations) can often be enhanced concurrently, thus allowing time for internal protective factors that lower suicide risk to be reestablished. As noted earlier, Brent et al. (1991) showed that guns in the home, even when locked or stored separately from ammunition, were associated with firearms suicide. Simon (2007) proposed that protection against gun suicides can be enhanced by designating a willing, responsible family member or other third party who would remove all guns from the home, car, or workplace, separate the ammunition, and secure the guns in a place outside the home where they are unknown to the patient. The designated responsible person then calls the clinician or designee to confirm that the gun safety management plan has been properly executed, before the patient is discharged.

Ordinarily, family and community support are important protective factors, but this cannot be assumed. For inpatients, interviews are essential to determining family members' capacity to provide genuine support. Psychoeducation and referral to community mental health programs can provide treatment continuity and "connectedness." Following a brief inpatient hospital stay, some patients will maintain a positive transference to the institution that can be a protective factor against suicide.

Experience teaches clinicians that a therapeutic alliance with the patient is a protective factor, although no evidence-based research supports this clinical consensus. Clinicians are shocked and bewildered when a patient with whom they believed a therapeutic alliance existed attempts or completes suicide between outpatient sessions. Like all protective factors, the therapeutic alliance does not afford absolute protection. It can be influenced by many factors beyond the clinician's knowledge or control. Moreover, the therapeutic alliance may not develop during short length of hospital stays, in limited outpatient sessions, or during brief, infrequent medication management appointments. Thus, the clinician may place unwarranted reliance on an assumed therapeutic alliance.

The suicide prevention contract has gained wide acceptance, although no studies demonstrate that it is an effective protective factor in preventing suicide (Stanford et al. 1994). When utilized as a substitute for competent suicide risk assessment, it can become a suicide risk factor.

Conclusion

No suicide risk management is complete without thorough assessment of protective factors. Protective factors that are identified require close scrutiny. Having a family may not necessarily be protective. Families, like individuals, may be dysfunctional and unsupportive of the patient. Mobilization of protective factors is an essential aspect of treatment and safety management of the suicidal patient.

KEY CLINICAL CONCEPTS

- A dynamic interplay exists between risk and protective factors.
- Protective factors should be systematically assessed, as are suicide risk factors.
- Any protective factor(s) can be overcome by the severity of the patient's mental illness.
- General evidence-based protective factors should alert the clinician to inquire about whether the patient has any uniquely individual protective factors.
- Restoring and enhancing protective factors form an essential therapeutic intervention for the patient at risk for suicide.

References

Borowsky IW, Ireland M, Resnick MD: Adolescent suicide attempts: risks and protectors. Pediatrics 107:485–493, 2001

Brent DA, Perper JA, Allman CJ, et al: The presence and accessibility of firearms in the homes of adolescent suicide: a case control study. JAMA 266:2989–2995, 1991

Dervic K, Oquendo MA, Grunebaum MF, et al: Religious affiliation and suicide attempt. Am J Psychiatry 161:2303–2308, 2004

Fawcett J: Depressive disorders, in The American Psychiatric Publishing Textbook of Suicide Assessment and Management. Edited by Simon RI, Hales RE. Washington, DC, American Psychiatric Publishing, 2006, pp 255–275

Fawcett J, Shefter W, Clark D, et al: Clinical predictors of suicide in patients with major affective disorders: a controlled prospective study. Am J Psychiatry 144:35–40, 1987

Linehan MM, Goodstein JL, Nielsen SL, et al: Reasons for staying alive when you are thinking of killing yourself: the Reasons for Living Inventory. J Consult Clin Psychol 51:276–286, 1983

Lizardi D, Currier D, Galfalvy H, et al: Perceived reasons for living in index hospitalization and future suicide attempt. J Nerv Ment Dis 195:451–455, 2007

Malone KM, Oquendo MA, Hass GL, et al: Protective factors against suicidal acts in major depression. Am J Psychiatry 157:1084–1088, 2000

Marzuk PM, Tardiff K, Leon AC, et al: Lower risk of suicide during pregnancy. Am J Psychiatry 154:122–123, 1997

Oquendo MA, Dragatsi D, Harkavy-Friedman J, et al: Protective factors against suicidal behavior in Latinos. J Nerv Ment Dis 193:438–443, 2005

Resnick PJ: Recognizing that the suicidal patient views you as an adversary. Curr Psychiatry 1:8, 2002

Shenassa ED, Rogers MI, Spalding KI, et al: Safer storage of firearms at home and risk of suicide: a study of protective factors in a nationally representative sample. J Epidemiol Community Health 58:841–848, 2004

Simon RI: Gun safety management with patients at risk for suicide. Suicide Life Threat Behav 37:518–526, 2007

Stanford EJ, Goetz RR, Bloom JD: The No Harm Contract in the emergency assessment of suicide risk. J Clin Psychiatry 55:344–348, 1994

Veeveers JE: Parenthood and suicide: an examination of a neglected variable. Soc Sci Med 7:135–144, 1973

CHAPTER 4

Behavioral Risk Assessment of the Guarded Suicidal Patient

PSYCHIATRISTS and other mental health professionals are trained to assess patients by direct observation and examination. Observational data can identify behavioral suicide risk factors that inform treatment and safety management, thus avoiding total reliance on patient reporting.

Identification of behavioral suicide risk factors is an important component in the systematic suicide assessment of all patients at risk. Patients evaluated in the emergency department or admitted to the psychiatric unit are often at heightened risk for suicide. Time is of the essence in busy emergency rooms and on inpatient units where lengths

Adapted with permission from Simon RI: "Behavioral Risk Assessment of the Guarded Suicidal Patient." *Suicide and Life-Threatening Behavior* 38:517–522, 2008.

of stay are short. Behavioral risk factors can facilitate early identification of the guarded suicidal patient.

A search of Google, Google Scholar, PsycINFO, Cochrane Library, PubMed, Medline, Ovid, CINAHL (Cumulative Index to Nursing and Allied Health Literature), and ERIC databases, using the following search terms and their variations, "behavioral suicide risk assessment" and "guarded suicidal patient," yielded no results.

The Guarded Suicidal Patient

Patients are often guarded and evasive in their initial and subsequent encounters with a psychiatrist or other mental health professional, without necessarily having the conscious intent to deceive the clinician. For example, some patients are initially frightened, embarrassed, denying, minimizing, and defensive. The Chronological Assessment of Suicide Events (CASE) approach is a practical interviewing strategy for eliciting valid suicide ideation, especially with the guarded suicidal patient (Shea 1998). The guarded, deceptive suicidal patient, however, intentionally attempts to conceal active suicidal ideation, intent, or plan from the clinician (Simon 2006b). The patient who is determined to complete suicide views the psychiatrist or mental health professional as an enemy (Resnick 2002).

Isometsa et al. (1995) found that the majority of patients who completed suicide did not communicate their suicide intent during their final appointment. In a retrospective study of 76 inpatient suicides, Busch et al. (2003) indicated that 77% of the patients denied suicidal ideation in their last recorded communication. Approximately 25% of patients at risk for suicide do not admit suicidal ideation to clinicians but do tell their families (Fawcett et al. 1993). A study by Robins (1981) of 134 suicides showed that 69% communicated suicide intent to a spouse and 50% to a friend, but only 18% to a mental health professional, within 12 months of suicide.

Patients at high risk for suicide often communicate their suicide intent only to the most important persons in their lives, but not necessarily to the psychiatrist, even after direct questioning (Fawcett et al. 1990). However, patients at mild to moderate risk for suicide usually communicate their intent to physicians or to other family members. The majority of patients who commit suicide do not communicate their intent during their last therapeutic appointment (Isometsa et al. 1995).

The assessment of the guarded suicidal patient should include, when possible, input from significant others. If the patient refuses to provide authorization, the clinician can still call and just listen, without revealing confidential information about the patient, unless the patient withholds consent for any contact with others. In some instances, an emergency exception to confidentiality may exist (Simon and Shuman 2007). Moreover, the Health Insurance Portability and Accountability Act of 1996 (HIPAA) permits psychiatrists and other "health care providers" who are treating the same patient to communicate without expressed permission from the patient (45 Code of Federal Regulations §164.502).

The guarded patient may admit to having had suicidal intentions prior to being evaluated but denies it during his or her evaluation. Some guarded patients deny being suicidal, even though other sources of information indicate that the patient is at high risk for suicide (e.g., emergency room evaluation, treaters, hospital transfer records, significant others, police). Although not directly observed by the clinician, classic behavioral suicide risk factors, such as the patient making a will, giving away valuable possessions, placing his or her life in order, or leaving a suicide note, may be described by significant others.

If there is sufficient time, routine psychological testing and suicide scales can be helpful in assessing the guarded suicidal patient. Sullivan and Bongar (2006, p. 193) caution that "[s]uicidal ideation and elevated suicide risk are often present in patients whose initial presentation may not trigger a suicide inquiry." They also observe that "patients often disclose more information regarding suicidal thoughts and behaviors on self-report measures than during clinical interviews."

A common aim of the deceptive, guarded suicidal patient is to avoid hospitalization or to obtain an early release from the hospital. When confronted with involuntary hospitalization, the guarded suicidal patient may sign a voluntary admission form but then aggressively press for an early discharge. Some guarded suicidal patients elope or sign out against medical advice. Once they leave the hospital, they attempt or complete suicide.

Evidence-Based Behavioral Risk Factors for Suicide

Evidence-based behavioral suicide risk factors can be arranged according to a hierarchy of evidence (Table 4–1). Systematic reviews (meta-analysis) are the highest level of evidence, followed by cohort studies (prospective), and case-control studies (retrospective) of risk (Gray 2004). Table 4–1 lists behavioral suicide risk factors along with supporting studies. Non-evidence-based behavioral suicide risk factors are derived from case reports and case series, and, lastly, from clinical opinion and clinical consensus. Clinical opinion and clinical consensus are important in suicide risk assessment, especially when combined with evidence-based studies.

Assessing Behavioral Suicide Risk Factors

Assessing behavioral risk factors informs the clinician's initial and ongoing treatment and management of the guarded suicidal patient. Several of the behavioral suicide risk factors listed in Table 4–1 are responsive to treatment and management. Behavioral suicide risk factors not only apply to the inpatient psychiatric unit but also to other clinical settings (e.g., emergency room, outpatient).

Deliberate self-harm is frequently a visible suicide behavioral risk factor with a high association with suicide attempts or completions (Cooper et al. 2005; Hawton and Harris 2007). Fawcett et al. (1987) identified "short-term" suicide risk factors derived from a 10-year prospective study of 954 patients with major affective disorders that were statistically significant for suicide within 1 year of assessment. The observable risk factors included psychic anxiety, diminished concentration, global insomnia, and depressive turmoil (agitation). Irritability often observed in patients with major depressive disorder is also correlated with depression severity and suicide attempts (Perlis et al. 2005). In a systematic review, Hansen (2001) found that akathisia, often confused with agitation, was not associated with increased suicide risk.

Agitation is a sentinel behavioral risk factor. Fawcett (2007, p. 670) provides the following excellent description of agitation: "Agitation can frequently be estimated by observing the patient fidgeting, wringing hands, moving, picking while seated, or at more severe levels by pacing, moaning or pounding doors and walls all the way to assaulting behavior." Agitation in extreme forms might look like extreme irritability but, generally, agitation shows more of a motor component (Jan Fawcett, M.D., personal communication, October 23, 2007).

TABLE 4–1. Behavioral suicide risk factors: hierarchy of evidence[a]

Systematic reviews (meta-analysis)

- Suicide attempts (Harris and Baraclough 1997)
- Substance abuse/intoxication (Harris and Baraclough 1997)
- Eating disorders (Harris and Baraclough 1997)
- Physical illness (Harris and Baraclough 1994)

Cohort studies

- Depression (Fawcett et al. 1990)
- Manic and mixed states (Fawcett et al. 1990)
- Psychosis (Warman et al. 2004)
- Panic attacks (Fawcett et al. 1990)
- Anxiety (Fawcett et al. 1987)
- Agitation/irritability (Fawcett et al. 1990; Perlis et al. 2005)
- Global insomnia (Fawcett et al. 1990)
- Melancholic features (Grunebaum et al. 2004)
- Symptom severity (Murphy et al. 1992)
- Diminished concentration (Fawcett et al. 1990)
- Hopelessness (Beck et al. 1990)
- Deliberate self-harm (Cooper et al. 2005; Hawton and Harris 2007)

Case-control studies

- Violent threats or behaviors (Connors et al. 2001)
- Impulsive aggression (Dumais et al. 2005)
- Physical illness, elderly (Quan et al. 2002)

Case reports or case series

- Akathisia (case reports)
- Isolation/inpatient (Simon and Gutheil 2002)
- Absence of therapeutic alliance/inpatient (Simon and Gutheil 2002)

TABLE 4–1. Behavioral suicide risk factors: hierarchy of evidence[a] *(continued)*

Clinical opinion or clinical consensus

- Individual "signature" suicide risk behaviors
- Absence of treatment alliance
- Concealment of lethal objects
- Suicide rehearsal
- Nonadherence to treatment
- Signing out against medical advice
- Elopement attempt
- Contemporaneous suicide note

---

[a]Observable behaviors and conditions.

Harris and Barraclough (1997), in a systematic review, determined the standardized mortality ratio (SMR) for psychiatric disorders. The SMR is a determination of the relative risk of suicide for a particular disorder compared with the expected rate of suicide in the general population. Psychiatric disorders with the highest SMR included eating disorders, affective disorders, substance abuse, and schizophrenia. A psychiatric diagnosis can sometimes be inferred from the behavioral presentation of the patient (e.g., anorexia, catatonia, mania). At the initial assessment of the guarded suicidal patient, the clinician may observe behaviors associated with a diagnosis. Diagnostic clarity, however, is often difficult to achieve. Behaviors may be associated with one or more diagnoses. For example, agitation may be observed in schizophrenia, bipolar disorder, major depression, anxiety disorders, and other diagnoses.

Some patients may have individualized "signature" behaviors that are associated with the risk of suicide; for example, a schizophrenic patient who stuttered would be at increased risk of suicide when he stopped stuttering (Simon 2004). Similarly, an obsessive patient would display an annoying hum when at increased risk for suicide. However, no psychiatric studies identify stuttering or humming as risk factors for suicide. Only the clinician with a thorough knowledge of the patient can discover such highly reliable suicide risk factors.

No single behavioral risk factor in Table 4–1 is, by itself, pathognomonic for attempted or completed suicide. *Pattern recognition* of behavioral suicide risk factors is necessary. For example, a sudden, unexplained improvement in the patient at high risk for suicide may reflect a deep sense of peace or even happiness, based on a final decision to complete suicide (e.g., the "smiling" suicidal patient). Nonetheless, in such a case, the behavioral suicide risk factor pattern usually remains unchanged, belying the rapid improvement.

Case Example

A 38-year-old, severely depressed physician is admitted to a psychiatric unit after he purchased a gun and left a suicide note for his wife stating, "Please forgive me. I have finally found the peace and happiness I always craved." He is placed on one-to-one arm's length safety precautions.

The patient remains seclusive, "cheeks" his medications, and avoids staff and other patients. On the second day of hospitalization, he fashions a noose from bed sheets (rehearsal). When confronted by staff, the patient states, "I just want to get my wife's attention." He gives the same reason for leaving a suicide note. Despite recent marital turmoil, his wife remains supportive, but the patient is indifferent to her visits. The patient continues to deny suicide ideation, intent, or plan. He remains severely depressed, agitated, and unable to sleep. His demeanor exhibits hopelessness and despair. The patient is placed on constant visual observation by the staff after being assessed at high risk for suicide.

On the fifth day of hospitalization, the patient's mood and agitation improve, but his appetite and sleep have not improved. He takes medication reluctantly and has not developed a therapeutic alliance with the psychiatrist or the clinical staff. Based on improved mood and decreased agitation, the patient's observation level is reduced to 15-minute checks. A few hours later, his roommate discovers the patient attempting to hang himself with a bed sheet and calls to the staff. The patient sobs, "All I want is peace. Let me die!" He is placed again on one-to-one arm's length safety precautions and reevaluated.

Is the sudden or rapid improvement of a patient at high risk for suicide genuine or is it feigned? In the Case Example, the patient is feeling relief because of his decision to complete suicide. The patient displayed a sudden improvement in mood and agitation, without a substantial improvement in other behavioral risk factors.

Behavioral assessment is not a substitute for a systematic assessment of suicide risk and protective factors that encompasses clinical, interpersonal, situational, and statistical (demographic) dimensions (Simon 2006b). The behavioral risk assessment should be integrated into a systematic suicide assessment when more information about the patient becomes available.

Inpatients

The admission of guarded patients at high risk for suicide, combined with brief hospital lengths-of-stay, makes rapid behavioral risk assessment essential for initial treatment and management decisions. Simon and Gutheil (2002) described a recurrent behavioral pattern observed on the inpatient unit in which the guarded suicidal patient is withdrawn, usually nonadherent to the treatment plan, pressing for early discharge, staying in the hospital room, and avoiding unit activities. The guarded suicidal patient readily agrees to a suicide prevention contract—even signing such a document if it is proffered. The patient tries to avoid the psychiatrist and unit staff. He or she is amazingly adept at "disappearing" on the psychiatric unit, especially when the psychiatrist arrives.

Observable protective factors include adherence to treatment, engagement with staff and other patients, and participation in unit activities (e.g., group therapies). The guarded suicidal patient may "play the game," superficially cooperating with the staff to obtain an early release from the hospital and to complete suicide. Protective factors, if present, may not become fully evident until additional history is obtained from collateral sources (e.g., significant others, treaters, treatment records).

It may not be possible to determine the level of suicide risk (low, moderate, high) of a guarded patient based solely on behavioral risk factor assessment. The purpose of behavioral suicide risk assessment is to identify and treat the guarded patient at high risk for suicide in time-limited situations (e.g., emergency room, psychiatric inpatient unit, outpatient settings). Behavioral risk factors are assessed in the "here-and-now." They are essential components of real time, formal suicide risk assessment. No evidence-based research identifies "short-term" or "imminent" risk factors that can predict when, or even if, a patient will attempt or complete suicide (Simon 2006a).

Emergency Patients

The guarded suicidal patient presents special assessment problems for the emergency room (ER) physician and the crisis counselor. The guarded patient vehemently denies suicidal ideation, suicide intent, or a suicide plan. While in the ER, the patient may be able to conceal most, if not all, behavioral suicide risk factors. Family members or police who accompany the patient to the ER often describe behavioral risk factors that necessitated bringing the patient to the ER.

If the ER patient is receiving outpatient treatment, the patient's therapist may not be available to provide essential clinical information to the ER clinician, especially during the early morning hours, when suicide crises frequently occur. Behavioral suicide risk assessment can assist the clinician make admission or discharge decisions from the ER, especially when information about the patient is sparse. For example, individuals seen in the ER who are seeking hospital admission for shelter and food often declare that they are "suicidal," but do not demonstrate discernible behavioral suicide risk factors. They are often unaccompanied.

Outpatients

An outpatient at risk for suicide may deny suicide intentions because of fear that the clinician may seek hospitalization. Unlike the inpatient clinician who is assisted by the treatment team, the outpatient clinician is often hampered by having had a limited number of sessions with the patient and less opportunity to observe the patient or receive reports from others. Although the clinician providing long-term outpatient treatment "knows" the patient, observation of behavioral suicide risk factors is largely limited to the therapy sessions. The psychiatrist who sees a patient briefly and infrequently for medication management has the least opportunity to observe behavioral risk factors, even though he or she is no less responsible for assessing the patient's risk for suicide (Meyer and Simon 2006). In split-treatment arrangements, close collaboration with treating therapists regarding patients' risk for suicide should be standard practice.

Conclusion

Assessing behavioral suicide risk factors is an essential component of systematic suicide risk asssessment. Most psychiatric disorders have accompanying behavioral symptoms that can assist clinicians in assessing the guarded suicidal patient. Behavioral assessment is not a substitute for systematic suicide risk assessment. Collateral sources of information must be obtained.

KEY CLINICAL CONCEPTS

- Observational data can be used to identify behavioral suicide risk factors that inform treatment and safety management, thus avoiding total reliance on patient reporting.

- Identification of behavioral suicide risk factors is an important component in systematic suicide assessment of all patients at risk.

- Behavioral risk factors can facilitate early identification of the guarded, deceptive suicidal patient.

- Patients may disclose more information about suicidal thoughts and behaviors on self-report measures than during the clinical interview. However, self-report measures should not displace competent suicide risk assessment.

- The assessment of the guarded suicidal patient should include, when possible, input from significant others.

References

Beck AT, Brown G, Bercheck RJ, et al: Relationship between hopelessness and ultimate suicide: a replication with psychiatric outpatients. Am J Psychiatry 147:190–195, 1990

Busch KA, Fawcett J, Jacobs DG: Clinical correlates of inpatient suicide. J Clin Psychiatry 64:14–19, 2003

Connors KR, Cox C, Duberstein PR, et al: Violence, alcohol, and completed suicide: a case control study. Am J Psychiatry 158:1701–1705, 2001

Cooper J, Kapur N, Webb R, et al: Suicide after deliberate self-harm: a 4-year cohort study. Am J Psychiatry 162:297–303, 2005

Dumais A, Lesage AD, Alda M, et al: Risk factors for suicide completion in major depression: a case control study of impulsive and aggressive behaviors in men. Am J Psychiatry 162:2116–2124, 2005

Fawcett J: Comorbid anxiety and suicide in mood disorders. Psychiatr Ann 37:667–671, 2007

Fawcett J, Scheftner WA, Clark DC, et al: Clinical predictors of suicide in patients with major affective disorders: a controlled prospective study. Am J Psychiaty 144:35–40, 1987

Fawcett J, Scheftner WA, Fogg L, et al: Time related predictors of suicide in major affective disorders: a controlled study. Am J Psychiatry 147:1189–1194, 1990

Fawcett J, Clark DC, Busch KA: Assessing and treating the patient at risk for suicide. Psychiatr Ann 23:244–255, 1993

Gray GE: Concise Guide to Evidence-Based Psychiatry. Washington, DC, American Psychiatric Publishing, 2004

Grunebaum MF, Galfalvy HC, Oquendo MA, et al: Melancholia and the probability and lethality of suicide attempts. Br J Psychiatry 184:534–535, 2004

Hansen L: A critical review of akathisia, and its possible association with suicidal behaviour. Hum Psychopharmacol 16:495–505, 2001

Harris EC, Barraclough BM: Suicide as an outcome for medical disorders. Medicine 73:281–286, 1994

Harris CE, Baraclough B: Suicide as an outcome for mental disorders. Br J Psychiatry 170:205–228, 1997

Hawton K, Harris L: Deliberate self-harm in young people: characteristics and subsequent mortality in a 20-year cohort of patients presenting to hospital. J Clin Psychiatry 68:1574–1583, 2007

Health Insurance Portability and Accountability Act of 1996 (HIPAA) [PL 104–191, 110 Stat 1936], 1996

Isometsa ET, Heikkinen ME, Martunen MJ, et al: The last appointment before suicide: is suicide intent communicated? Am J Psychiatry 152:919–922, 1995

Meyer DJ, Simon RI: Split treatment, in The American Psychiatric Publishing Textbook of Suicide Assessment and Management. Edited by Simon RI, Hales RE. Washington, DC, American Psychiatric Publishing, 2006, pp 235–251

Murphy GE, Wetzel RD, Robbins E, et al: Multiple risk factors predict suicide in alcoholism. Arch Gen Psychiatry 49:459–463, 1992

Perlis RH, Fraguas R, Fava M, et al: Prevalence and clinical correlates of irritability in major depressive disorder: a preliminary report from the Sequenced Treatment Alternatives to Relieve Depression study. J Clin Psychiatry 66:159–166, 2005

Quan H, Arboleda-Florez J, Fick GH, et al: Association between physical illness and suicide among the elderly. Soc Psychiatry Psychiatr Epidemiol 37:190–197, 2002

Resnick PJ: Recognizing that the suicidal patient views you as an adversary. Curr Psychiatr 1:8, 2002

Robins E: The Final Months: Study of the Lives of 134 Patients Who Committed Suicide. New York, Oxford University Press, 1981

Shea SC: Chronological assessment of suicide events: a practical interviewing strategy for the elicitation of suicidal ideation. J Clin Psychiatr 59 (suppl 20):58–72, 1998

Simon RI: Assessing and Managing Suicide Risk: Guidelines for Clinically Based Risk Management. Washington, DC, American Psychiatric Publishing, 2004

Simon RI: Imminent suicide: the illusion of short-term prediction. Suicide Life Threat Behav 36:296–301, 2006a

Simon RI: Suicide risk: assessing the unpredictable, in The American Psychiatric Publishing Textbook of Suicide Assessment and Management. Edited by Simon RI, Hales RE. Washington, DC, American Psychiatric Publishing, 2006b, pp 1–32

Simon RI, Gutheil TG: A recurrent pattern of suicide risk factors observed in litigated cases: lessons in risk management. Psychiatr Ann 32:384–387, 2002

Simon RI, Shuman DW: Clinical Manual of Psychiatry and Law. Washington, DC, American Psychiatric Publishing, 2007

Sullivan GR, Bongar B: Psychological testing in suicide management, in The American Psychiatric Publishing Textbook of Suicide Assessment and Management. Edited by Simon RI, Hales RE. Washington, DC, American Psychiatric Publishing, 2006, pp 177–196

Warman DM, Forman E, Henriques GR, et al: Suicidality and psychosis: beyond depression and hopelessness. Suicide Life Threat Behav 37:77–86, 2004

CHAPTER 5

Psychiatric Disorders and Suicide Risk

IN the United States, more than 90% of suicides are associated with mental illness (Harris and Barraclough 1997). Psychiatric diagnosis is an important—if not the most important—suicide risk factor. Every psychiatric disorder except mental retardation is associated with suicide risk (Table 5–1). Mann et al. (1999) proposed the stress-diathesis model of suicide behavior. For suicide to occur, a trigger (mental illness) and a preexisting vulnerability to suicide behaviors must be present.

Major depressive disorder, bipolar disorder, schizophrenia, and substance abuse disorder are associated with high suicide risk (American Psychiatric Association 2003). In the Harris and Barraclough (1997) study, eating disorders had the highest standardized mortality ratio (SMR). Franko and Keel (2006) found high rates of suicide in patients with anorexia nervosa. Suicide rates were not as elevated with bulimia nervosa.

Patients with personality disorders are at seven times greater risk for suicide than the general population (Harris and Barraclough 1997; see Chapter 1, "Suicide Risk Assessment: A Gateway to Treatment and Management"). Cluster B personality disorders, especially borderline

TABLE 5–1.   **Mental and physical disorders and mortality**

Disorder	SMR[a]
Eating disorders	23.14
Major depression	20.35
Sedative abuse	20.34
Mixed drug abuse	19.23
Bipolar disorder	15.05
Opioid abuse	14.00
Dysthymia	12.12
Obsessive-compulsive disorder	11.54
Panic disorder	10.00
Schizophrenia	8.45
Personality disorders	7.08
AIDS	6.58
Alcohol abuse	5.86
Epilepsy	5.11
Child and adolescent disorders	4.73
Cannabis abuse	3.85
Spinal cord injury	3.82
Neuroses	3.72
Brain injury	3.50
Huntington's chorea	2.90
Multiple sclerosis	2.36
Malignant neoplasms	1.80
Mental retardation	0.88

[a]Standardized mortality ratio (SMR) is calculated by dividing observed mortality by expected mortality.
Source.   Adapted from Harris CE, Barraclough B: "Suicide as an Outcome for Mental Disorders." *British Journal of Psychiatry* 170:205–228, 1997.

and antisocial personality disorders, place patients at increased risk for suicide (Duberstein and Conwell 1997). Cluster B traits and impulsive aggression represent significant risk factors for suicide (McGirr et al. 2009). Unemployment, financial problems, family discord, and interpersonal conflicts and loss increase suicide risk in persons with personality disorders (Heikkinen et al. 1997).

Individuals with narcissistic traits or personality disorder are vulnerable to "shame suicides" when faced with intolerable humiliation arising from events such as scandals, business failures, or criminal charges (Simon 2004). The diagnostic criteria for personality disorders are not as robust as those for Axis I mental health disorders. Semistructured assessment instruments can support but not take the place of clinical assessment. The diagnosis of a personality disorder usually requires a series of interviews, in contrast to Axis I disorders, which can often be diagnosed at the initial evaluation. When performing an initial multiaxial psychiatric evaluation of the patient, clinicians often record Axis II as "deferred."

Under Axis III physical disorders, the following conditions are associated with increased risk of suicide: AIDS, epilepsy, spinal cord injury, brain injury, Huntington's chorea, and cancer (American Psychiatry Association 2003). Other physical illnesses associated with increased risk include head and neck malignancies, peptic ulcer disease, systemic lupus erythematosus, chronic hemodialysis-treated renal failure, heart disease, prostate disease, and chronic obstructive pulmonary disease.

Short hospital lengths-of-stay; 30-minute initial evaluations, followed by 10-minute "med checks" in split-treatment settings where psychiatrist and therapist neither know nor call each other. Limited numbers of psychotherapy sessions often do not provide sufficient time for the clinician to make the diagnosis of personality disorders. The clinician should, whenever possible, review prior treatment records and/or make calls to former or current treaters. These measures may reveal the diagnosis of a preexisting personality disorder. The clinician must spend sufficient time with the patient to develop a diagnosis and differential diagnosis.

Comorbidity

Comorbid psychiatric diagnoses increase suicide risk (Henriksson et al. 1993). Most common comorbidities include major depression, borderline and antisocial personality disorders, and alcohol and other substance abuse disorders. Psychiatric comorbidity is an important risk factor for suicide attempts in patients with borderline personality disorder, especially depression (Black et al. 2004). Patients with major depression and generalized anxiety disorder had high levels of suicidal ideation compared with depressed patients without generalized anxiety disorder (Zimmerman and Chelminski 2003). In this study, 93% of patients who committed suicide had one or more Axis I diagnoses. Severe depression and anxiety combined markedly elevate suicide risk. Isometsa et al. (1996) found that all individuals with a personality disorder who had committed suicide had received at least one Axis I diagnosis. A diagnosis on Axis II was made in 31% of cases, and at least one diagnosis on Axis III was made in 46% of cases.

Kessler et al. (1999), in a population survey of 5,877 individuals, found a dose-response relationship between the number of disorders and suicide attempts. The total number of disorders, not the types of disorders, was determinative. Regarding suicide risk assessment, careful attention should be given to all current and past psychiatric diagnoses as well as current Axis III physical conditions and disorders.

DSM-IV-TR Specifiers and Suicide Risk

DSM-IV-TR (American Psychiatric Association 2000) provides severity and course specifiers for a number of psychiatric disorders, including major depressive disorder, single episode, and severe with melancholic features. Severity specifiers are mild, moderate, and severe. The course specifiers are in partial or full remission or prior history. The depressive episode can be either single or recurrent. Melancholic feature specifier criteria are available.

Suicide risk increases proportionately with illness severity reflected in the level of treatment (American Psychiatric Association 2003). Whether major depression is a single episode or recurrent episodes also has significance for suicide risk. In younger patients, suicides tend to occur early in the illness course (Hoyer et al. 2000). Recurrent major depression entails serious suicide risk. Major depression recurs in 40%–50% of cases (Spijker et al. 2002). With each recurrence, severity and duration of illness may increase, and each recurrence tends to precede more frequent recurrences (Kendler et al. 2000). The depression can become more refractory to treatment. Hopelessness and demoralization, combined with loss of employment and impaired relationships, further elevate suicide risk. Feature specifiers such as psychosis or melancholia also add to suicide risk.

Diagnostic accuracy is essential to competent suicide risk assessment. Evaluation of specifiers (severity, course, features) provides additional important data regarding suicide risk, as discussed in the next section. Multiaxial psychiatric diagnosis identifies comorbidities among Axis I, II, and III; the assessment of stressors that are present in patients at risk for suicide (Axis IV); and the level of functional impairment, with its psychological, social, and occupational dimensions.

Suicide Risk Associated With Melancholic Features of Major Depressive Disorder: An Example

Suicide risk is increased in patients with major depressive disorder with melancholic features compared with patients with major depressive disorder. Grunebaum et al. (2004) compared suicide attempts associated with melancholic versus nonmelancholic major depression in 377 patients who were consecutively enrolled in the depression protocols of two university hospitals. Of these, 151 participants (40%) met DSM-IV criteria for melancholia. The investigators found that melancholic patients had more serious suicide attempts and increased probability and lethality of future attempts. Patients without melancholia usually did not require psychiatric hospitalization as frequently as melancholic patients.

McGrath et al. (2008), using a STAR*D protocol, found that 23.5% of outpatients met the DSM-IV criteria for melancholic symptom features. These patients were significantly more likely than study participants without melancholic features to have made prior suicide attempts and were judged to be a suicide risk at the time of study entry. The finding that approximately one-quarter of patients with major depression met

DSM-IV specifier criteria for melancholic features is consistent with other studies (Khan et al. 2006). Study participants who met criteria for melancholic features demonstrated higher depression severity scores, greater Axis I comorbidity (mainly anxiety and substance use disorders), and a lower likelihood of remission rate with treatment by a selective serotonin reuptake inhibitor (SSRI).

Melancholia

Leventhal and Rehm (2005) found that melancholic depression is qualitatively different in symptomatology than nonmelancholic depression. The distinction is supported by biological ("endogenous") factors, personality traits, unresponsiveness to treatment, and increased risk of suicide. Khan et al. (2006) found that sociodemographic and other external factors usually are not as prominent as occurs with nonmelancholic depressed patients. They concluded that genetic or biological factors play an important role in the development of melancholic symptoms.

DSM-IV-TR lists the following specifier criteria for melancholic features:

A. Either of the following:
   • Loss of interest or pleasure in all, or almost all, activities
   • Lack of reactivity to pleasurable stimuli
B. Three (or more) of the following:
   • Distinct quality of mood (e.g., different from bereavement sadness)
   • Depression worse in the morning
   • Early morning awakening (at least 2 hours before usual awakening)
   • Marked psychomotor retardation or agitation
   • Significant anorexia or weight loss
   • Excessive or inappropriate guilt

DSM-IV-TR lists a number of clinical and biological markers associated with melancholic depression:

• Psychomotor changes nearly always present (observable)
• Less likely to have a premorbid personality disorder

- Less likely to have a clear precipitant
- Less likely to respond to a trial of placebo medication
- More frequent as inpatients than outpatients
- Less likely to occur in milder compared with more severe major depressive episodes
- More likely to occur in patients with psychotic features
- More frequently associated with laboratory findings:
  - Dexamethasone nonsuppression
  - Elevated cortisol concentrations in plasma, urine, and saliva
  - Alteration of sleep EEG profiles
  - Abnormal asymmetry on dichotic listening tasks

Suicide Risk

Next to eating disorders, major depression is the psychiatric disorder most frequently associated with suicide (Harris and Barraclough 1997). As noted, melancholic features substantially increase suicide risk (Grunebaum et al. 2004). Concurrent psychosis, comorbidity, and the lower likelihood of remission also increase the risk of suicide. McGrath et al. (2008) found that melancholic features were associated with significantly reduced remission following treatment with an SSRI.

The diagnosis of melancholic features can be missed for a variety of reasons. A lack of diagnostic rigor may not distinguish between melancholic and nonmelancholic depression. Moreover, clinicians may not consider the increased risk of suicide associated with melancholic features.

Clinical settings can also influence diagnosis. Shortened inpatient lengths of stay may not allow time for correct diagnosis, especially when clinicians treat patients for brief periods of time. In partial hospitalization programs, allied mental health professionals may not place sufficient emphasis on diagnosis, focusing more on patients' psychological dynamics and interpersonal relationships.

Melancholic patients are less frequently treated in outpatient settings. Thus, clinicians may have less experience in diagnosing this condition. Split treatment, in which the psychiatrist sees patients infrequently for only 10 or 15 minutes and a psychotherapist who provides therapy, may not allow for a sufficient time to make the correct diagnosis, even after an initial 45-minute or 1-hour evaluation. Moreover, the diagnosis of melancholic features may only become apparent over time. Close collaboration and communication between psychiatrist and therapist can facilitate accurate diagnosis (Simon 2004). All patients diagnosed with major depression should be carefully assessed for melancholic features.

The diagnosis of melancholic features can also be overlooked because of symptom overlap between melancholic and nonmelancholic core depression. Melancholia, as a specifier, does not have the categorical diagnostic clarity of a stand-alone psychiatric disorder. In addition, the A criteria of melancholic features (loss of pleasure in all, or almost all, activities, and lack of reactivity to usually pleasurable stimuli) are dimensional expressions of severe depression, whereas the B criteria are categorical. The core feature of melancholia is the severity of depression, a dimensional criterion that can be difficult to assess diagnostically.

Treatment and Management

The elevated suicide risk associated with melancholic patients requires accurate diagnosis, systematic suicide risk assessment, and evidence-based treatments. Melancholic patients respond more favorably to tricyclic antidepressants (TCAs) and monoamine oxidase inhibitors (MAOIs) than to SSRIs (Angst et al. 1993; Peselow et al. 1992). In addition, electroconvulsive therapy (ECT) is also indicated for the melancholic patient, especially if the patient is acutely suicidal and unresponsive to pharmacotherapy (American Psychiatric Association 2006; Kim et al. 2006). Some melancholic patients are responsive only to ECT.

If a patient diagnosed with major depressive disorder is not improving despite aggressive treatment, the diagnosis should be revisited to rule in or out melancholic features. With delay in treatment, the depression can become entrenched, resulting in the patient experiencing hopelessness, demoralization, and increased suicide risk. Delay may also adversely affect the patient's employment status and personal relationships.

Conclusion

In the United States, greater than 90% of suicides are associated with mental illness. While all psychiatric disorders except mental retardation carry an increased risk of suicide, melancholic features of major depressive disorder are associated with a higher risk of suicide. Standardized mortality ratios vary according to specific diagnoses. For example, eating disorders and major depression have the highest SMRs. Personality disorders have much lower SMRs. Comorbidity increases suicide risk according to the number of mental disorders. DSM-IV-TR specifiers further identify increased risk of suicide. Melancholic features of major depressive disorder are associated with a higher risk of suicide than major depression without melancholia. Diagnostic precision, with attention given to DSM-IV-TR specifiers, informs treatment and management of the patient at risk for suicide.

KEY CLINICAL CONCEPTS

- Every psychiatric disorder, with the exception of mental retardation, is associated with suicide risk.

- Psychiatric diagnosis is an important risk factor. Making the correct diagnosis is crucial.

- Comorbidity of Axis I, II, and III disorders increases the risk of suicide.

- It is important to consider DSM-IV-TR specifier criteria that may increase suicide risk associated with the psychiatric disorder.

- The clinician must spend sufficient time with the patient to acquire enough information for a reasonable diagnosis and differential diagnosis.

References

American Psychiatric Association: Diagnostic and Statistical Manual of Mental Disorders, 4th Edition, Text Revision. Washington, DC, American Psychiatric Association, 2000, pp 419–420

American Psychiatric Association: Practice guidelines for the assessment and treatment of patients with suicidal behaviors. Am J Psychiatry 160 (suppl 11):1–60, 2003

American Psychiatric Association Practice Guidelines for the Treatment of Psychiatric Disorders: Compendium 2006. Arlington, VA, American Psychiatric Association, 2006, p 800

Angst J, Scheidegger P, Stabl M: Efficacy of moclobemide in different patient groups. Results of new subscales of the Hamilton Depression Rating Scale. Clin Neuropharmacol 16 (suppl 2):S55–S62, 1993

Black DW, Blum N, Pfohl B, et al: Suicidal behavior in borderline personality disorder: prevalence, risk factors, prediction and prevention. J Pers Disord 18:226–239, 2004

Duberstein P, Conwell Y: Personality disorders and completed suicide: a methodologic and conceptual review. Clin Psychol Sci Pract 4:359–376, 1997

Franko DL, Keel PK: Suicidality in eating disorders: occurrence, correlates, and clinical implications. Clin Psychiatry Rev 26:769–782, 2006

Grunebaum MF, Galfalvy HC, Oquendo MA, et al: Melancholia and the probability and lethality of suicide attempts. Br J Psychiatry 184:534–535, 2004

Harris CE, Barraclough B: Suicide as an outcome for mental disorders. Br J Psychiatry 170:205–228, 1997

Heikkinen MD, Hendriksson MM, Isometsa ET, et al: Recent life events and suicide in personality disorders. J Nerv Ment Dis 85:373–381, 1997

Henriksson MM, Hillevi M, Aro MD, et al; Mental disorders and comorbidity in suicide. Am J Psychiatry 150:935–940, 1993

Hoyer EH, Mortensen PB, Olesen AV: Mortality and causes of death in a total national sample of patients with affective disorders admitted for the first time between 1973 and 1993. Br J Psychiatry 176:76–82, 2000

Isometsa ET, Henriksson MD, Heikkinen ME, et al: Suicide among subjects with personality disorders. Am J Psychiatry 153:667–673, 1996

Kendler KS, Thornton LM, Gardner CO: Stressful life events and previous episodes in the etiology of major depression in women: an evaluation of the "Kindling" hypothesis. Am J Psychiatry 157:1243–1251, 2000

Kessler RC, Borges G, Walters EE: Prevalence of and risk factors for life-threatening suicide attempts in the National Comorbidity Survey. Arch Gen Psychiatry 56:617–626, 1999

Khan A, Carrithers J, Preskorn SH, et al: Clinical and demographic factors associated with DSM-IV melancholic depression. Ann Clin Psychiatry 18:91–98, 2006

Kim HF, Marangell LB, Yudofsky SC: Psychopharmacological treatment and electroconvulsive therapy, in The American Psychiatric Publishing Textbook of Suicide Assessment and Management. Edited by Simon RI, Hales RE. Washington, DC, American Psychiatric Publishing, 2006, pp 199–220

Leventhal AM, Rehm LP: The empirical status of melancholia: implications for psychology. Clin Psychol Rev 25:5–44, 2005

Mann JJ, Waternaux C, Haas GL, et al: Toward a clinical model of suicidal behavior in psychiatric patients. Am J Psychiatry 156:181–189, 1999

McGirr A, Alda M, Séquin M, et al: Familial aggregation of suicide explained by cluster B traits: a three-group family study of suicide controlling for major depressive disorder. Am J Psychiatry 166:1124–1134, 2009

McGrath PJ, Khan AY, Trivedi MH, et al: Response to selective serotonin reuptake inhibitors (citalopram) in major depressive disorder with melancholic features: a STAR*D report. J Clin Psychiatry 69:1847–1855, 2008

Peselow ED, Sanfilipo MP, Difiglia C, et al: Metabolic/endogenous psychiatry. Am J Psychiatry 149:1324–1334, 1992

Simon RI: Assessing and Managing Suicide Risk: Guidelines for Clinically Based Risk Management. Washington, DC, American Psychiatric Publishing, 2004

Spijker J, deGraaf R, Bijl RV, et al: Duration of major depressive episodes in the general population: results from the Netherlands Mental Health Survey and Incidence Study. Br J Psychiatry 181:208–213, 2002

Zimmerman M, Chelminski I: Generalized anxiety disorder in patients with major depression: is DSM-IV's hierarchy correct? Am J Psychiatry 160:504–512, 2003

CHAPTER 6

Sudden Improvement in Patients at High Risk for Suicide

Real or Feigned?

A patient admitted for treatment to a hospital is expected to improve. But sudden clinical improvement in patients assessed as being at high risk for suicide poses a dilemma: is this a valid though rapid result of treatment, a decision to die that brings relief, or a deception aimed at rapid discharge? Moreover, is the patient glad, ambivalent, or disappointed about surviving a suicide attempt? Such a development challenges the psychiatrist's clinical acumen. Malpractice cases make clear the seriousness of the problem.

Typically, this conundrum arises on inpatient units, although it also occurs in other clinical settings. The psychiatrist and the treatment

Adapted with permission from Simon RI, Gutheil TG: "Sudden Improvement in High-Risk Suicidal Patients: Should It Be Trusted?" *Psychiatric Services* 60:387–389, 2009.

team must determine not only whether the suicidal patient's improvement is real or feigned, but also whether any improvement is durable enough to sustain the patient's safety after discharge.

The patient at high risk for suicide often makes a near-lethal suicide attempt prior to admission or even while on the psychiatric unit. Multiple suicide risk factors may be present; protective factors are minimally operative or absent.

The psychiatrist's approach to such patients is based on systematic suicide risk assessment. Complicating that assessment is the fact that the length of stay on most psychiatric inpatient units is brief: in some cases, 4–5 days or less. The usual treatment goal in such settings is rapid stabilization and reduction of suicide risk. Discharge planning begins at admission. Because the clinical focus is on returning psychiatric inpatients to the community as soon as possible, the patient at high risk for suicide who evinces sudden, unexpected improvement fits in all too well with this treatment model. Thus, the extent of the persisting risk can be easily overlooked.

Real Improvement

Many psychiatric inpatients at high risk for suicide do improve rapidly shortly after admission. Improvement can mean that the patient is no longer at acute high risk but remains at chronic high risk for suicide at discharge, requiring comprehensive postdischarge planning (see Chapter 7, "Patients at Acute and Chronic High Risk for Suicide: Crisis Management"). Patients at acute high risk for suicide cannot be expected to pose no risk at discharge. Most patients at moderate risk for suicide are treated as outpatients. The structured milieu, the initiation of treatment, the effects of medications, the safety measures provided, and the peer interactions can promote rapid improvement. Anti-anxiety, antipsychotic, and sleep medications can be effective within minutes or hours; a good night's sleep can result in rapid improvement in the patient's clinical condition. Apart from medications, psychosocial interventions—especially group therapy—decrease anxiety, reduce isolation, improve reality testing, provide needed support, and shorten the hospital length of stay (Simon 2004). Detoxifying substance abuse patients can reduce, often dramatically, high suicide risk.

The improving patient usually gives the staff permission to speak to persons who know the patient. This source of additional information may or may not corroborate the patient's account of illness. The treatment team observes whether the patient adheres to treatment recommendations and conforms to unit policies. The patient displays real improvement by attending group meetings, socializing with other patients, and being visible on the unit.

Most patients at high risk for suicide show gradual, often halting improvement. Real improvement can be rapid but is not often sudden and unexpected. Basic indices of improvement occur in sleep, appetite, symptom reduction, treatment adherence, and socialization. Real improvement is a process, even when rapid. Although the feigning suicidal patient will try to mimic real improvement, the imitation falls short of clinical credibility.

Feigned Improvement

Case Example

A married, middle-aged businessman, admitted with depression and suicidal preoccupations, is aloof and distant on the ward. In a short time, he begins to interact with staff and attend groups and occupational therapy, all indicia of improvement. Plans are made for his discharge. A team member expresses serious doubts about this plan, given that the patient told him in the middle of the previous night that he was still seriously desperate and hopeless. Confronted, the patient admits a plan to hang himself immediately after discharge. The discharge is canceled. After 2 weeks of treatment and adjustment of medication, the patient's halting improvement becomes genuine, and a discharge with prompt follow-up (e.g., partial hospitalization and psychiatrist appointment) is planned.

The patient at high risk for suicide who feigns improvement by denying suicide ideation, intent, or plan often displays contrary behaviors and attitudes that belie denials (Simon and Gutheil 2002). His or her true intent is to obtain release from the hospital as soon as possible, or to wait out a short length of stay, while planning to complete suicide shortly after discharge.

A near-lethal suicide attempt usually precedes inpatient admission or occurs on the psychiatric unit. As a measure of the seriousness of the suicide attempt, the patient will have left notes to family members, made a will, and put financial matters in order. It is not unusual for the patient to state that he or she is disappointed in not completing suicide. Once admitted, the patient may display a spectrum of signs—from subtle to overt—that indicates persisting suicidal intent, despite denials. Typical signs include disturbed eating and sleeping patterns that remain unchanged; averted gaze; and poor personal hygiene and disheveled appearance. The patient is isolative, spending most of the time in the room. He remains seclusive, with only minimal or superficial contact with the staff and other patients. The patient attends group therapy sporadically, participates minimally, or not at all. He refuses permission for the staff to speak with family members. At the time of admission, approximately 25% of patients at risk for suicide deny having suicidal ideation to the clinician but do tell their families (Robins 1981).

In addition, it is difficult for the psychiatrist and other members of the treatment team to form a therapeutic alliance, ordinarily a powerful protective factor against suicide, with the patient (Goldblatt and Schatzberg 1992; Havens 1967; Maltsberger 1986). Many psychiatric inpatients, even within a short length of stay, are able to form some level of therapeutic alliance with the clinical staff or hospital facility. Adherence to the medication regimen and to unit rules is tenuous in patients at risk. Medications, when taken, can energize the patient, creating the impression of improvement but without diminishing underlying hopelessness and suicide intent.

First-time-hospitalized, high-achieving, high-functioning, ambitious patients, who become depressed and are unable to work or to work productively, are often at high risk for suicide (Simon and Gutheil 2002). The reality of having a mental illness is mortifying. It is viewed as a personal failing and is experienced as a devastating narcissistic injury. Such patients, who are often professionals, are highly defined by their work. Before committing suicide, many of these previously high-functioning patients gradually withdraw from important relationships, much like patients who are terminally ill and are preparing to die. The patient's first hospitalization usually indicates the onset of severe depression and significant suicide risk. The patient applies considerable pressure on the clinician and unit staff for an immediate discharge, stating, "I don't belong here with these crazy people" or "I will lose my job and family if I stay here." Most mental health professionals are high functioning, making it easy to identify with such patients and to minimize their suicide risk.

When patients feign being "no longer suicidal," fundamental change does not occur in the severity of their clinical condition, behavior, and attitude. Although the patient may occasionally laugh, for example, while playing a game on the unit, he may be only momentarily distracted from depression, suicidal preoccupations, and intent. This levity should not be construed as improvement, in the absence of other clinical indicia of improvement. Feigned improvement is usually sudden and surprising. It is not a gradual process but an unexpected event that can occur at any point during inpatient hospitalization.

Suicide Risk Assessment

The patient who is determined to commit suicide considers the psychiatrist and clinical staff the enemy (Resnick 2002). They stand in the path of the patient's suicide intent. Tragic consequences can ensue from the simplistic assumption that every suicidal patient wants help and will cooperate with treatment. In addition, the absence of protective factors is an indication of continuing high suicide risk. Individual, "signature" risk factors, if known, can provide solid clinical guidance (e.g., the stuttering patient who, when at high risk for suicide, speaks clearly). The clinician must trust his or her suicide risk assessment, if not the patient. Initial blanket distrust of the patient will likely doom any hope for a therapeutic alliance. Finally, the therapeutic alliance may fail because of cultural differences and misunderstandings.

A situation frequently occurs in the emergency department, where a "patient" fakes being suicidal. The magic words, "I am suicidal," open the door to hospitalization, food, and shelter. Unless systematic suicide risk assessment is performed, once on the psychiatric unit, the faking sick patient behaves much the same as the patient faking well. For example, the patient does not cooperate with inpatient policies, remains seclusive, and is noncompliant with treatment recommendations. Unlike the faking-well suicide patient, he attempts to extend his hospital stay.

A clinical distinction should be made between the guarded and the deliberately deceptive suicidal patient (see Chapter 4, "Behavioral Risk Assessment of the Guarded Suicidal Patient"). Patients are frequently guarded or evasive during their initial encounter with the psychiatrist and staff. Guarded patients may not necessarily have the conscious intent to deceive the clinician. For example, some patients are frightened, embarrassed, denying, minimizing, and defensive rather than consciously deceptive.

When the clinician is conducting suicide risk assessments, behavioral risk factors should be included (Simon 2008). Behavioral risk factors associated with suicide speak louder than the deceptive patient's words. Table 6–1 contains evidence-based behavioral suicide risk factors that do not require a patient's cooperation to assess. For example, the behavioral manifestations of most psychiatric disorders are usually readily observable. Also, all psychiatric disorders, with the exception of mental retardation, have accompanying suicide risk potential (Harris and Barraclough 1997).

Gathering information from collateral sources is basic to competent suicide risk assessment of high-risk suicide patients who suddenly improve. Family members are critical sources of information. When the patient refuses to authorize discussion with family members, the clinician can obtain valuable information by just listening without revealing confidential information. However, some patients refuse to authorize any contact with significant others. Under Health Insurance Portability and Accountability Act of 1996 (HIPAA) regulations, physicians can communicate with other physicians without obtaining the patient's prior consent.

In emergencies, the psychiatrist may need to obtain critical information from collateral sources. He or she can try to persuade but not coerce the patient to authorize release of information. Ethically, it is permissible to breach confidentiality in order to protect the suicidal patient (American Psychiatric Association 2001). The emergency exception to obtaining consent is another available option. The clinician should be knowledgeable about federal and state statutes and the courts that define "medical emergency" either narrowly or expansively (Simon 2004). Prior treatment records, especially discharge summaries from other hospitals, cannot usually be obtained quickly, but calls or e-mails to previous treaters may provide critical clinical information about the patient on an urgent basis. With the ubiquity of pagers and cell phones, most clinicians can be reached quickly. A doctor's call is usually responded to without delay. In an emergency situation, such as when a clinician is treating a high-risk suicidal patient, an exception to maintaining confidentiality exists both ethically and legally (Simon and Shuman 2007).

The treatment team is an essential source of patient information 24 hours a day, 7 days a week. The multidisciplinary team has a "thousand eyes." The patient's current psychiatric record must be read care-

---

TABLE 6–1.   Some behavioral suicide risk factors

- Suicide attempt
- Psychiatric diagnosis[a]
- Substance abuse/intoxication
- Eating disorder
- Physical illness
- Depression
- Melancholic features
- Manic and mixed states
- Psychosis
- Anxiety
- Agitation/irritability
- Global insomnia
- Symptom severity
- Diminished concentration
- Violent threats or behaviors
- Impulsivity/aggression

---

[a]Observable manifestations.
Source.   Adapted with permission from Simon RI: "Behavioral Risk Assessment of the Guarded Suicidal Patient." *Suicide and Life-Threatening Behavior* 38:517–522, 2008.

fully. It inevitably contains vital behavioral and other information regarding the patient's risk for suicide (Simon and Hales 2006).

Iatrogenic sudden improvement ("miraculous insurance cures") occurs when the clinician inflates the patient's suicide risk on admission or subsequently to obtain additional hospital stay days. If the insurance benefits are not approved, the patient suddenly "improves" and is discharged. This situation is fraught with liability risk if the patient attempts or commits suicide. A malpractice claim may be filed for negligent discharge.

When a patient is determined to commit suicide at the earliest opportunity, an apparently "real" improvement in his clinical condition may occur. For example, "mood lightening" occurs, falsely reassuring the staff that the patient is improving. Medications are taken as prescribed; social isolation ceases; and the patient attends and participates in group therapy and other unit activities. However, the patient's desire to die and escape psychic pain remains unchanged.

The core symptoms of a psychiatric disorder usually remain unchanged. For example, the vegetative symptoms of depression will persist. In psychotic patients, thought disorder, hallucinations, and delusions continue to lurk behind the patient's sham improvement. The patient may continue to restrict access to collateral sources of information. And lethal implements may be secreted in the patient's room or elsewhere on the unit.

Psychiatric inpatients present along a dynamic continuum of truthfulness and deception, making it difficult to discern real from feigned improvement at any given time and in any given circumstance. A common form of deception occurs when inpatients minimize their symptoms to gain off-unit smoking privileges. Clear and unambiguous examples of real versus feigned improvement among high-risk suicidal patients previously described are found only at the poles of the continuum. Because many inpatients improve rapidly and are discharged, the high-risk suicidal patient's specious improvement can be very difficult—and, on occasion, impossible—to distinguish from real improvement. Consultation may help discern real from feigned improvement. The clinician should "never worry alone" (T.G. Gutheil, personal communication, 2008).

Risk Management

The risk management problem posed by sudden unexpected improvement and consequent suicide is captured in this excerpt from an actual deposition in a case where suicide occurred:

> Q: Have you ever heard the term "mood lightening?"
> A: Yes.
> Q: And what is your understanding as to what that means?
> A: That once the person has decided that they are going to commit suicide, that sort of like a burden has been lifted, and they're more comfortable.
> Q: And it manifests itself in what appears to be a better mood on the part of the patient?
> A: Yes.
> Q: And mood brightening is *a sign and symptom of potential suicidality?* [emphasis added]
> A: Yes.

As should be made clear from this excerpt, the clinician's problem is distinguishing expected and desired improvement from signs of the decision to die. From a risk management viewpoint, the critical variables are the presence of consistent signs of improvement absent the contradictory signs listed in Table 6–1 and a consistency of the clinical picture of the patient to all observers. If the patient's progress presents any ambiguity about the process just noted, changes in level of observation should probably be delayed to allow more extensive data gathering.

Because clinicians are human, even the most careful analysis may fail. The subtlety of the signs of suicidal intent may simply preclude their detection. On the other hand, patients genuinely improving may nevertheless show sleep disturbance, agitation, or group avoidance for reasons other than suicidal intent. Because informed clinical judgment is the only viable resource for making such subtle distinctions (as well as representing the antithesis of negligence), the treater's clinical reasoning and suicide risk assessments must be carefully documented.

In the usual inpatient setting, the psychiatrist typically rests at the top of a pyramid of staff. This implies both a pyramid of decision making (final decisions) and of observational data (the psychiatrist as final common pathway for information). Regrettably, psychiatrists do not always review the entire chart or attend sufficiently to staff input. Even more regrettably, some psychiatrists assume that only what the patient tells the psychiatrist is true or important, discounting information from other team members.

Most clinicians are familiar with patients who put on a "smiley face" when speaking to the doctor but let their guard down with other team members and admit their underlying despair, as in the Case Example. This kind of selective candor also resembles how family members may be taken into the patient's confidence and may not hear the persisting depression or suicidal intent. Such a familiar situation requires the team leader to pay close attention to the observations of staff, who have usually seen the patient not for a few minutes, but for an entire shift.

Some clinicians may prefer to employ a variety of standardized measures such as the Beck Hopelessness Scale, Hamilton Rating Scale for Depression (see Chapter 10, "Suicide Risk Assessment Forms: Clinician Beware"), or similar instruments. These measures cannot substitute for systematic suicide assessment, but their use may at least attest to the clinician's efforts to deepen understanding of the patient and constitute an argument against negligence. Standard practice, however, does not require that routine use of standardized measures be employed in the assessment of suicide risk. "Know thy patient" is the imperative measure.

Conclusion

The suicidal patient "faking good" is very difficult to identify when patients are hospitalized for brief stays. Improvement bias expects patients to stabilize quickly. For the most part this happens. But the problem remains regarding how well do we know the patient. The focus of attention following psychiatric admission quickly shifts to discharge planning. The feigning suicidal patient does not have long to wait for discharge.

KEY CLINICAL CONCEPTS

- Spend sufficient time with the patient to do an adequate psychiatric evaluation and suicide risk assessment.

- Obtaining patient information from collateral sources is critical in short length-of-stay hospitalizations.

- Sudden improvement, also known as "mood lightening," can result from the patient's resolve to complete suicide.

- Psychiatric inpatients are expected to improve quickly during a short length of stay. Thus, feigned improvement may be overlooked.

- Real improvement of the high-risk suicidal patient is a process, even when it occurs quickly. Feigned improvement is an event.

- Behavioral risk factors help the clinician to assess suicide risk in the guarded or dissimulating patient.

References

American Psychiatric Association: Principles of Medical Ethics With Annotations Especially Applicable to Psychiatry. Washington, DC, American Psychiatric Association, 2001

Goldblatt M, Schatzberg A: Medication and the suicidal patient, in Suicide and Clinical Practice (Clinical Practice 21). Edited by Jacobs D. Washington, DC, American Psychiatric Press, 1992, pp 23–41

Harris CE, Barraclough B: Suicide as an outcome for mental disorders. Br J Psychiatry 170:205–228, 1997

Havens LL: Recognition of suicidal risks through the psychologic examination. N Engl J Med 276:210–215, 1967

Health Insurance Portability and Accountability Act of 1996 (HIPAA) [PL 104–191, 110 Stat 1936], 1996

Maltsberger JT: Suicide Risk: The Formulation of Clinical Judgment. New York, New York University Press, 1986

Resnick PJ: Recognizing that the suicidal patient views you as an adversary. Curr Psychiatr 1:8, 2002

Robins E: The Final Months: Study of the Lives of 134 Persons Who Committed Suicide. New York, Oxford University Press, 1981

Simon RI: Assessing and Managing Suicide Risk: Guidelines for Clinically Based Risk Management. Washington, DC, American Psychiatric Publishing, 2004

Simon RI: Behavioral risk assessment of the guarded suicidal patient. Suicide Life Threat Behav 38:517–522, 2008

Simon RI, Gutheil TG: A recurrent pattern of suicide risk factors observed in litigated cases: lessons in risk management. Psychiatr Ann 32:384–387, 2002

Simon RI, Hales RE (eds): The American Psychiatric Publishing Textbook of Suicide Assessment and Management. Washington, DC, American Psychiatric Publishing, 2006

Simon RI, Shuman DW: Clinical Manual of Psychiatry and Law. Washington, DC, American Psychiatric Publishing, 2007

PART II

MANAGEMENT

CHAPTER 7

Patients at Acute and Chronic High Risk for Suicide

Crisis Management

ALTHOUGH the acute and chronic high-risk suicidal patient is a categorical paradigm, the severity of suicide risk is dimensional and dynamic, affected by constantly changing risk and protective factors. No bright line separates chronic from acute high suicide risk. Suicide risk factors, such as depression and hopelessness, often overlap in patients at acute and chronic high risk for suicide.

The transition from chronic to acute can be gradual and nuanced or alarmingly rapid. O.R. Simon et al. (2001), in a case-control study of 153

Portions of this chapter adapted with permission from Simon RI: *Assessing and Managing Suicide Risk: Guidelines for Clinically Based Risk Management.* Washington, DC, American Psychiatric Publishing, 2004.

case subjects, found that 24% spent less than 5 minutes between the decision to attempt suicide and the actual, near-lethal attempt. In the gradual transition from chronic to acute high risk, early identification may allow for aggressive treatment and management. Knowing the patient's evolving symptoms, the prodromal "signature" suicide risk-factor profile, preceding a prior attempt(s) can alert the clinician to take quick action.

The patient at chronic high risk for suicide bears a certain similarity to the cardiac patient at chronic high risk for a heart attack. For example, the high-risk cardiac patient has hypertension, obesity, hypercholesterolemia, angina or prior heart attack, diabetes, and a family history of cardiovascular disease. If the patient has an acute myocardial infarction, which requires emergency intervention, and survives, the patient's status usually reverts to chronic high risk for another acute cardiac event, even after appropriate treatment.

A patient at chronic high risk for suicide can become acutely suicidal for a number of reasons, including resurgence of the psychiatric illness, nonadherence to medication, resumption of substance abuse, stressful life events, and loss of protective factors. These factors can rapidly propel the patient from chronic high-risk status into acute high-risk status. Emergency treatment may return the patient to chronic high-risk status. For example, a severely depressed patient at acute, high risk for suicide, whose adequate medication trials have failed, may respond quickly to electroconvulsive therapy (ECT) with a reduction in depression and suicide risk.

The term *acute* describes the intensity (severity) and magnitude (duration) of the symptom. For example, sleeplessness can vary in severity from early-morning waking to debilitating global insomnia; duration can range from moments of hopelessness to unrelenting hopelessness in a depressed suicidal patient (Fawcett 2006). A high-risk factor is supported by an evidence-based association with suicide. Once a patient is determined to be at acute, high risk for suicide, immediate clinical intervention is required to prevent suicide. Some patients remain at high risk for suicide for periods of hours, days, weeks, or a few months (Fawcett 2006).

Patients at chronic, high risk for suicide have acute suicidal crises requiring emergency care. They are at risk for suicide over years, usually requiring long-term preventive treatment to reduce suicide risk and relapses. Patients at acute, high risk for suicide display commonly occurring state-related risk factors (Table 7–1).

TABLE 7–1.   Acute high suicide risk factors

- Severe symptoms of psychiatric disorder
- Suicidal ideation
- Recent and past suicide attempts
- High lethality of current suicide attempt
- Substance abuse
- Hopelessness
- Global insomnia
- Panic attacks
- Agitation/mixed states (bipolar I or II)
- Comorbid anxiety and depression
- Painful physical condition or illness
- Recent loss

Note.   There is no single pathognomonic suicide risk factor.

Patients who are chronically at high risk for suicide present with commonly occurring trait-related risk factors (see Table 7–2). Chronic (static) risk factors may include, for example, a family history of suicide, prior attempts, childhood abuse, and a history of impulsive behaviors. As noted previously, suicide risk factors often overlap in acute and chronic high-risk suicidal patients.

Clinicians in outpatient office practice often have the opportunity to work with the patient over time, gathering data crucial to decision making regarding the patient who develops a high risk for suicide. Clinicians in emergency departments and inpatient units often do not have the same time advantage for clinical understanding of the acute, high-risk patient who walks in off the street. In this situation, clinicians must be able to conduct and trust the suicide risk assessments that guide their clinical decision making.

Clinical Management

The treatment and management of the acute or chronic high-risk suicidal patient is a daunting clinical challenge. Most psychiatrists in clinical practice have encountered or will encounter these patients. Every

---

TABLE 7–2. **Chronic high risk suicide factors**

- History of suicide attempts (high lethality)
- Previous hospital admissions
- Cluster B, Axis II disorders
- Alcohol/substance abuse
- Impulsivity/aggression (self and/or others)
- Parasuicidal behaviors
- Comorbidity (Axis I and Axis II)
- History of child physical/sexual abuse
- Family history of suicide attempts and completions
- Family history of mental disorders
- Chronic physical pain
- Persistent hopelessness
- Chronic Axis I and Axis II disorders
- Recurrent depression
- Interpersonal loss

Note. Suicide risk factors often overlap in patients at acute and chronic high risk for suicide (e.g., depression, hopelessness).

---

case presents clinical nuances and differences that cannot be encompassed by a definitive set of management guidelines. General principles, however, are illustrated in the following case example, which presents treatment and management issues in an outpatient setting. Emergency department and psychiatric inpatient unit staffs, however, have the most frequent contact with high-risk suicidal patients. Clinicians practicing in the emergency department and inpatient unit usually have more experience treating acute, high-risk suicidal patients. They tend to receive more clinical, psychological, and physical support from other mental health professionals than outpatient clinicians (Simon 2004).

Case Example

A psychiatrist has been treating a 35-year-old, single woman for 4 years, providing both psychotherapy and medication management. The patient's current diagnoses are Axis I major depressive disorder, severe, recurrent, and generalized anxiety disorder; and Axis II borderline personality disorder. The patient was initially hospitalized at age 17, after impulsively slashing her wrists. Severed tendons required surgical repair. She had two subsequent brief hospitalizations for near-lethal overdoses. The diagnosis each time was major depressive disorder, severe, recurrent. At each hospitalization, the patient admitted unrelenting suicidal ideation with a specific plan. The last hospitalization occurred 2 years ago, following a rejection by a male friend. The patient's family is supportive, as are a number of friends.

The patient was sexually abused at age 8 years. Her mother was treated for depression. An uncle committed suicide. The patient has worked steadily as a librarian. Her relationships with men have been fraught with unreasonable demands, followed by feelings of rejection. Bouts of alcohol abuse have accompanied severe depression.

Until recently, the patient's depression and anxiety responded to antidepressant medication. She has a working alliance with the psychiatrist that becomes frayed during a crisis. The current, severe depression and anxiety followed loss of her job due to workplace cutbacks. The patient is abusing alcohol again, feeling hopeless, and has intense suicide ideation with a plan to jump from a nearby bridge. She also describes insomnia and irritability. The patient has not made a recent suicide attempt.

The psychiatrist recommends immediate hospitalization, but the patient adamantly refuses. Suicide risk assessment confirms that the patient has rapidly moved from chronic-high to acute-high suicide risk. The psychiatrist is faced with two options: immediate involuntary hospitalization or continuation of outpatient treatment. The patient's refusal of voluntary hospitalization is initially managed as a treatment issue. Asked why she has accepted hospitalization in the past under similar circumstances but now refuses, the patient replies that the loss of her job has been an essential source of self-esteem and stability. She says the loss is unbearable.

The psychiatrist now considers the risks and benefits of involuntary hospitalization but feels such a course of action would doom the doctor-patient relationship, leaving the patient bereft of a life-stabilizing relationship. Moreover, the patient will likely be discharged from involuntary hospitalization after a few days. This would further exacerbate her illness and suicide risk. The state civil commitment standard for involuntary hospitalization requires that the patient be at "imminent" risk of harm to self or others. This would be a difficult argument to make, given that the patient is continuing to see her psychiatrist.

The psychiatrist considers the risks and benefits of the outpatient option. He determines that the therapeutic alliance, though attenuated, supports the plan. A phone consultation is obtained with a colleague who agrees with the outpatient option. The treating psychiatrist recommends that the patient be seen more frequently, her medications adjusted, and a formal consultation obtained. The patient reluctantly agrees.

The family provides support, as in past hospitalizations. The psychiatrist feels that the patient's family is a crucial protective factor. The family joins the patient in a therapy session where a "We are in it together" strategy is implemented. Family members (parents, older brother, and sister) are asked to be aware of symptom changes, which should prompt a call to the psychiatrist. They are not asked to maintain a 24-hour vigil, which is unrealistic. The patient or family can reach the psychiatrist by cell phone. The patient agrees to partial hospitalization, with which she is familiar. The appointment is scheduled for the day after discharge. The psychiatrist will see the patient briefly each day, but longer, if necessary. A therapist trained in providing dialectical behavior therapy (DBT), with whom the patient has consulted in the past for suicide ideation, agrees to see the patient for brief, crisis therapy. Regular phone contact will be maintained between psychiatrist and therapist. The psychiatrist informs the patient that if the acute suicidal crisis continues despite intensive treatment, the option of hospitalization will be revisited. As a last resort, the psychiatrist knows that if the patient remains unimproved after a few days and again refuses hospitalization, the psychiatrist must pursue involuntary hospitalization. After a week of intensive treatment, the patient's depression and anxiety symptoms gradually improve. The patient reverts to chronic, high suicide risk status, as her acute suicide risk factors abate. The DBT will continue. The psychiatrist maintains careful, detailed documentation throughout the patient's suicide crisis, especially suicide risk assessment and his clinical decision-making rationale.

Commentary

To hospitalize or not to hospitalize, that is the conundrum that psychiatrists often face with high-risk suicidal patients. The decision is considerably more complicated when the need for hospitalization is clear but the patient refuses the recommendation. The decisions that the psychiatrist makes at this point are crucial for treatment and risk management.

Voluntary hospitalization is often a straightforward matter. The psychiatrist, after systematic suicide risk assessment, determines that the patient is at a level of suicide risk that requires hospitalization. As in the Case Example, the risks and benefits of continuing outpatient treatment are weighed against the risks and benefits of hospitalization.

If the patient agrees, arrangements are made for immediate hospitalization. The patient must go *directly* to the hospital, accompanied by responsible persons. The patient should not stop to do errands, get clothing, or make last-minute arrangements. A detour can provide the patient with the opportunity to attempt or complete suicide. If the patient is driven to the hospital, a safety locking mechanism under the sole control of the driver may prevent the patient from jumping out of the car. In some instances, psychiatrists have accompanied the patient to the hospital. However, psychiatrists have no legal duty to assume physical custody of the patient (*Farwell v. Un* 1990).

If the patient disagrees with the psychiatrist's recommendation for hospitalization, the refusal should be addressed as a treatment issue. Often, the need for hospitalization is acute; thus, a prolonged inquiry is not permitted. In addition, the therapeutic alliance may become strained. It is this clinical situation that tries the professional mettle of the psychiatrist. Consultation and referral are options for the clinician to consider, if time and the patient's condition allow. In the Case Example, the psychiatrist calls a colleague for a brief phone consult. The psychiatrist should never worry alone. Sleepless nights benefit neither the psychiatrist nor the patient.

The psychiatrist may decide not to hospitalize a patient who is assessed to be at moderate to high suicide risk. Protective factors may allow continuing outpatient treatment. In such a case, a good therapeutic alliance will be present, the psychiatrist will have worked with the patient for some time, and family support will be available. The psychiatrist will determine that the patient's suicide risk can be managed by more frequent visits and treatment adjustments. Also, supportive family members can help by providing observational data but should not be asked to provide 24-hour, eyeball-to-eyeball supervision of the patient (see Chapter 8, "Safety Management of the Patient at Risk for Suicide: Coping With Uncertainty"). Protective factors can be overwhelmed by a severe mental illness. In contrast, a patient assessed as being at moderate risk for suicide may need hospitalization when protective factors are few or are absent.

The psychiatrist may determine that the patient at high risk for suicide who refuses hospitalization does not meet the substantive criteria for involuntary hospitalization. For example, the criteria may contain the requirement that the patient must have made a suicide attempt within a specified period of time. The psychiatrist's options are to continue to treat the patient and deal with the issue of hospitalization as a treatment matter; see the patient more frequently; adjust medications; obtain consultation; reexamine the therapeutic alliance; consider an adjunctive, intensive outpatient program; refer the patient; or all of these. The referral option may not be feasible until the patient's current suicide crisis has passed. Frustration and anger with the suicidal patient can lead to abandonment of the patient (see Chapter 11, "Imminent Suicide, Passive Suicidal Ideation, and Other Intractable Myths").

Involuntary hospitalization should be utilized as an emergency clinical intervention, not as a defensive tactic to avoid malpractice liability or to provide a legal defense against a malpractice claim. Unnecessary hospitalization can worsen a patient's psychiatric condition and damage trust, which is important for future treatment. Although state civil commitment statutes vary, the substantive legal criteria for involuntary hospitalization generally include severe mental illness and/or dangerousness to self or others and the inability to provide for basic needs (Table 7–3). Commitment statutes do not require involuntary hospitalization of patients but are permissive

Psychiatrists have serious concerns about disrupting the patient's therapy by instituting involuntary hospitalization. Involuntary hospitalization also may jeopardize the patient's occupation and personal relationships. However, little or no therapeutic alliance exists when the acutely mentally ill patient who is at high risk for suicide refuses hospitalization. Discomfort or reluctance to involuntarily hospitalize a suicidal patient based on the psychiatrist's belief that it is coercive may lead to avoidance of a necessary hospitalization. The compelling clinical issues for the psychiatrist are patient treatment and safety. The psychiatrist must be prepared to take a firm but clinically supportive stand, if involuntary hospitalization is necessary. Ultimately, whatever decision is made should be the result of a reasoned clinical judgment.

In some localities, when the patient requires involuntary hospitalization, meaningful psychiatric hospitalization does not exist. The patient will likely be discharged within a few days from an overcrowded institution that grudgingly must accept another suicidal patient. Moreover, the patient's outpatient treatment may end without the goal of hospitalization having been achieved, thus creating the potential for tragedy. As in the Case Example, the psychiatrist may justifiably decide to treat the patient as an outpatient, in addition to making appro-

---

TABLE 7–3. Typical substantive and miscellaneous criteria for civil commitment

---

Substantive criteria

- Mentally ill
- Dangerous to self or others
- Unable to provide for basic needs

Miscellaneous criteria (in conjunction with one or more of the criteria above)

- Gravely disabled (unable to care for self, resulting in likely self-harm)
- Refusing hospitalization
- In need of hospitalization
- Danger to property
- Lacks capacity to make rational treatment decisions
- Hospitalization represents least restrictive alternative

Note. Criteria are statutorily determined, varying from state to state.
Source. Reprinted with permission from Simon and Shuman 2007.

priate adjustments in the treatment plan. Consultation in such a case is advisable. The psychiatrist should carefully document suicide risk assessments and the decision-making process.

Familiarity with state commitment laws and the availability of community emergency mental health services are necessities when suicidal crises arise. A patient may be civilly committed only when statutorily mandated criteria are met. Some clinicians labor under the mistaken assumption that they commit the patient when signing certification papers. Civil commitment (involuntary hospitalization) is a judicial decision. The court or an administrative body may agree or disagree with the clinician's recommendation to involuntarily hospitalize the patient.

Familiarity with available emergency mental health resources enables the clinician to act decisively. For example, many communities have mobile crisis units that can assist the involuntary hospitalization process. If a high-risk suicidal patient runs out of the office or emergency department when confronted by involuntary or even voluntary hospitalization, the police or mobile crisis unit can be called. The mobile crisis unit can petition for involuntary hospitalization, but it does not take custody of the patient, which the police can do. Police willingness to assist is dictated by their training and the availability of psychiatric facilities. Police assistance varies among jurisdictions.

The fear of being sued can adversely influence the psychiatrist's clinical judgment about involuntary hospitalization. The most common ground for a lawsuit involving involuntary hospitalization is the claim of wrongful commitment, giving rise to a cause of action for false imprisonment. Other theories of liability include assault and battery, malicious prosecution, abuse of process, and the intentional infliction of emotional distress. However, the risk of being sued for involuntary hospitalization is low. Once the decision to involuntarily hospitalize the patient is made, the psychiatrist should try to discuss the reasons with the patient in order to help preserve trust for future treatment.

States have provisions in the commitment statutes granting psychiatrists and other mental health professionals immunity from liability when they use reasonable clinical judgment and act in good faith (Simon and Shuman 2007). When the psychiatrist is petitioning for involuntary hospitalization, willful, blatant, or gross failure to follow statutory commitment procedures will not meet the good-faith provision. A malpractice suit for involuntary hospitalization of a patient is unlikely when an adequate examination is performed, statutory requirements are followed, and the certification is free of malice.

Statutory commitment laws, as noted previously, are permissive, leaving the decision of whether to involuntarily hospitalize a patient to the discretion of the mental health professional (Appelbaum et al. 1989). However, malpractice suits alleging failure to involuntarily hospitalize patients at risk for suicide have been filed against psychiatrists. A suit against a psychiatrist for failure to involuntarily hospitalize a patient is far more common than a lawsuit for certifying a patient. Careful documentation of suicide risk assessment, combined with the risk-benefit analyses for and against involuntary hospitalization, represents good clinical care and also provides a solid legal defense.

Circumstances may arise in which the psychiatrist feels uncertain about involuntary hospitalization as the best clinical option for a patient at acute, high risk for suicide. A tension exists between the patient's rights and the clinician's duty to treat. The medical model is outcome-driven, with a focus on patient and societal benefit. Civil libertarians express concern that *the ends* of preventing suicide may not justify *the means* of involuntary hospitalization. Involuntary hospitalization is justified if it appears likely that the patient will receive treatment and benefit from hospitalization (Stone 1976). Psychiatrists rely on their training and clinical experience to determine the best treatment disposition for their patients. When involuntary hospitalization is sought, the courts usually temper clinical biases through legal scrutiny in making the final decision.

The psychiatrist must not use the threat of involuntary hospitalization to coerce a suicidal patient into accepting treatments or procedures when he or she has no intention of petitioning for commitment. Persuasion engages the patient's reasoning ability to arrive at a desired goal. Coercion circumvents the patient's ability to reason and is undermined by manipulation (Malcolm 1992). When confronted with involuntary hospitalization, many patients opt for voluntary admission.

Involuntary hospitalization is a valid clinical intervention that may prevent suicide for appropriate patients. Looking back, involuntarily hospitalized patients may understand the necessity for hospitalization. Some patients are appreciative of the care they received (Gove and Fain 1977; Spensley et al. 1980).

Discharging High-Risk Patients

Discharge planning begins at admission and is refined during the patient's inpatient stay. Before the patient is discharged, a final post-discharge treatment and aftercare plan is necessary (see Table 7–4). Following discharge, suicide risk increases when the intensity of treatment is decreased (Appleby et al. 1999).

The patient's willingness to cooperate with discharge and aftercare planning is a critical determinant in establishing contact with follow-up treaters. The psychiatrist and treatment team structure the follow-up plan so as to encourage compliance. For example, psychotic patients at risk for suicide, who have a history of stopping their medications immediately on discharge, may be given a long-acting intramuscular neuroleptic that will last until they reach aftercare. Patients with comorbid drug and alcohol abuse disorders are referred to agencies equipped to manage dual-diagnosis patients.

Patients require education about their mental disorders. Family members should be similarly educated, when appropriate. One of the goals of educating patients about their disorders is to encourage adher-

---

TABLE 7–4.   Discharge planning for inpatients at risk for suicide

Risk-benefit analysis for both discharge and continued hospitalization

- Conduct systematic suicide risk assessments.
- Review patient's course of hospitalization: What is different about the patient's illness and life situation at the time of discharge?
- Spend sufficient time to have an adequate clinical understanding of the patient.
- Determine that patient has acclimated to therapeutic milieu, with sufficient time to develop meaningful relationships.
- Check whether sufficient time has elapsed to effectively evaluate the response to treatment.
- Arrange for patients at chronic risk for suicide to be seen in outpatient treatment soon after discharge.
- Consider a second opinion for difficult discharge decisions.
- Initiate gun safety management plan.

Support

- Determine whether patient is physically and emotionally able to obtain help.
- Inform patient of available mental health services.
- Determine whether support from family members or significant others is present.

Status of illness

- Evaluate what symptoms remain unchanged that can be effectively treated as outpatient.
- Ensure that patient receives psychoeducation regarding illness.
- Construct a workable discharge plan formulated in collaboration with patient.

Medication adherence

- Reinforce importance of adherence with medication treatment.
- Discuss with patient whether current side effects can be tolerated and managed outside hospital.

Therapeutic alliance

- Assess patient's capacity to work with mental health professionals.

Source.   Adapted from Simon and Shuman 2007.

ence to treatment and aftercare recommendations. Patients and their families often complain that they were not told their diagnosis or educated about treatment.

Limitations exist on the ability of psychiatrists to ensure follow-up treatment, a fact that must be acknowledged by both the psychiatric and the legal communities (Simon 1998). Beyond stabilization of the patient, the psychiatrist's options in bringing about positive changes may be limited or nonexistent. Also, the patient's failure to adhere to postdischarge plans and treatment often results in rehospitalization, hopelessness, and greater suicide risk. Psychiatric patients at moderate or moderate-to-high risk for suicide are increasingly treated in outpatient settings. It is the responsibility of the psychiatrist and treatment team to competently hand off the patient to appropriate inpatient aftercare. With the patient's permission, the psychiatrist or social worker should call the follow-up agency or therapist before discharge to provide information about the patient's diagnosis, treatment, and hospital course.

Follow-up appointments should be made as close to the time of discharge as possible. The psychiatrist presented in the case example earlier in this chapter is clearly familiar with the research regarding postdischarge suicide, which often occurs on the first day after discharge (Mehan et al. 2006). He schedules an appointment with partial hospitalization for the next day following discharge. The patient should have an actual appointment in-hand, or the attending psychiatrist or hospital clinician may need to provide an interim follow-up appointment. Encouraging patients to make their own appointments, while still in the hospital, fosters independent functioning. However, some patients at discharge are too disorganized to make their own appointments. The patient should know whom to call or where to go if an emergency arises before the first outpatient appointment. Homeless patients at risk for suicide should be placed in aftercare programs where follow-up is maximized. Consistent follow-up may not be possible for transient homeless patients. This limitation should be documented in the discharge note.

If the patient is being transferred to another facility, the assessment of the patient's current condition, including the patient's risk for suicide, should be communicated to the staff at the new facility. Written communication may be necessary: whenever possible, direct telephone conversations (duly documented) with the new treaters may be more effective in communicating information about the patient. In a phone call, questions can be asked and explanations given. The failure to provide relevant information to treaters who may be unaware of the suicide risk of a transferred patient can create liability problems for the psychiatrist. Abstracts from the psychiatric record and discharge summary should be forwarded to the postdischarge treater in a timely manner.

Most discharges involve a complex process that must be tailored to the patient's individual treatment needs and circumstances. The decision to discharge a patient is often more difficult than the decision to admit the patient. A risk-benefit assessment at discharge weighs the risks and benefits of continued hospitalization versus the risks and benefits of discharge. A number of factors need to be considered and weighed in the risk-benefit assessment, such as the discharge suicide risk assessment, the patient's severity of illness, the likelihood of compliance with follow-up care, the availability of family or other support, and the presence of a substance abuse disorder or other comorbid conditions. Documentation is essential.

The following are the two related critical questions to be asked in a risk-benefit assessment:

1. Has the patient improved sufficiently to function outside the hospital, or is this discharge doomed to fail?
2. What is different about the patient's condition or life situation at the time of discharge?

In a study of inpatient suicide, Fawcett et al. (2003) reported that "78% of the patients denied suicidal ideation or intent as their last communication" (p. 18). When a patient denies suicidal ideation or intent, systematic suicide risk assessment can help identify other clinical correlates of suicide risk.

A well-reasoned, clearly documented risk-benefit note that explains the psychiatrist's decision making at the time of discharge will help preempt second-guessing by a court, if the patient attempts or commits suicide and a lawsuit is filed. Assessing the risk of suicide is a "here and now" determination. Patients who are no longer at acute high risk for suicide often remain at chronic high-risk. The discharge note should indicate the acute suicide risk factors that have abated or remitted and the chronic (long-term) suicide risk factors that remain. The discharge note must also address the patient's chronic vulnerability to suicide. For example, the patient may become acutely suicidal again, depending on a number of factors, including the nature and cause of the psychiatric illness, adequacy of future treatment, extent of adherence to treatment recommendations, and unforeseeable life vicissitudes. Suicidal behaviors are the result of dynamic, complex interaction among a variety of clinical, personality, social, and environmental factors whose relative importance varies across time and situations.

Conclusion

The treatment and management of patients with acute and chronic high risk of suicide is a daunting clinical challenge. The patient at chronic high risk of suicide who is being treated as an outpatient and becomes acutely suicidal presents the clinician with difficult choices. Can the patient continue to be safely treated as an oupatient? If not, will the patient accept voluntary hospitalization, or must the patient be involuntarily hospitalized? Malpractice claims alleging failure to involuntarily hospitalize the acute high risk suicidal patient who attempts or completes suicide are relatively common.

The patient at acute and chronic high risk of suicide who is hospitalized also presents the clinician with difficult decisions regarding discharge. Careful discharge planning is required. Transition to oupatient treatment must be tailored to the clinical needs of the patient and the available community resources. The patient may require appointments with outpatient treaters the day after discharge, if possible. Litigation claiming negligent discharge is unfortunately common.

KEY CLINICAL CONCEPTS

- The severity of suicide risk is dimensional and dynamic, constantly governed by changing risk and protective factors. Thus, suicide risk assessment is a process, not an event.

- *Acute* describes the intensity (severity) and magnitude (duration) of symptoms; a high-risk factor is supported by an evidence-based association with suicide.

- No bright line separates chronic from acute high suicide risk. The transition from chronic to acute can be gradual and nuanced or alarmingly rapid. A patient's current evolving symptoms and suicide risk profile often display the symptoms and suicide risk profile of prior suicide crises or attempt(s), thus alerting the clinician to take quick action to prevent a suicide.

- Patients at chronic high risk for suicide can shift to acute high-risk status, secondary to both internal and external stressors, such as progression of illness, nonadherence to psychiatric treatment, or interpersonal loss.

- Patients at acute high risk for suicide usually display a number of state-related risk factors. Patients who are chronically at high risk for suicide often display a number of trait-related and static risk factors. But overlapping symptoms and risk factors are invariably present between acute and chronic high risk suicidal patients.

References

Appelbaum PS, Zonana H, Bonnie R, et al: Statutory approaches to limiting psychiatrists' liability for the patients' violent act. Am J Psychiatry 146:821–828, 1989

Appleby L, Dennehy JA, Thomas CS, et al: Aftercare and clinical characteristics of people with mental illness who commit suicide; a case control study. Lancet 353:1397–1400, 1999

Farwell v Un, 902 F 2d 282 (4th Cir 1990)

Fawcett J: Depressive disorders, in The American Psychiatric Publishing Textbook of Suicide Assessment and Management. Edited by Simon RI, Hales RE. Washington, DC, American Psychiatric Publishing, 2006, pp 255–275

Fawcett J, Clark DC, Busch KA: Clinical correlates of inpatient suicide. J Clin Psychiatry 64:14–19, 2003

Gove WR, Fain T: A comparison of voluntary and committed psychiatric patients. Arch Gen Psychiatry 34:669–697, 1977

Malcolm JG: Informed consent in the practice of psychiatry, in The American Psychiatric Press Review of Clinical Psychiatry and the Law, Vol 3. Edited by Simon RI. Washington, DC, American Psychiatric Press, 1992, pp 223–281

Meehan J, Kapur N, Hunt I, et al: Suicide in mental health inpatients within 3 months of discharge. Br J Psychiatry 188:129–134, 2006

Simon OR, Swann AC, Powell KE: Characteristics of impulsive suicide attempts and attempters. Suicide Life Threat Behav 32 (suppl):49–59, 2001

Simon RI: Psychiatrists' duties in discharging sicker and potentially violent inpatients in the managed care era. Psychiatr Serv 49:62–67, 1998

Simon RI: Assessing and Managing Suicide Risk: Guidelines for Clinically Based Risk Management. Washington, DC, American Psychiatric Publishing, 2004

Simon RI, Shuman DW: Clinical Manual of Psychiatry and Law. Washington, DC, American Psychiatric Publishing, 2007

Spensley J, Edwards D, White E: Patient satisfaction and involuntary treatment. Am J Orthopsychiatry 50:725–727, 1980

Stone AA: Mental Health and Law: A System in Transition (Publ No ADM-6-176). Rockville, MD, National Institute of Mental Health, 1976

CHAPTER 8

Safety Management of the Patient at Risk for Suicide

Coping With Uncertainty

FOR clinicians involved in the safety management of patients at risk for suicide, the tension between providing safety and allowing freedom of movement creates uncertainty. Clinicians also experience dissonance between the need to provide adequate supervision for patients at risk for suicide and the denial of insurance coverage by third-party payers for these services. The only true certainty is that effective treatment and safety management of the suicidal patient require the clinician's full commitment of time and effort.

Adapted with permission from Simon RI: "Patient Safety Versus Freedom of Movement: Coping With Uncertainty," in *The American Psychiatric Publishing Textbook of Suicide Assessment and Management*. Edited by Simon RI, Hales RE. Washington, DC, American Psychiatric Publishing, 2006, pp. 423–439.

After careful assessment, the safety management of the patient at risk for suicide is an informed judgment call. The provision of absolute safety is obviously an impossible task. Patients who are determined to commit suicide will find a way. They view the clinician as their enemy (Resnick 2002). Deception and lack of patient cooperation complicate safety assessments (see Chapter 4, "Behavioral Risk Assessment of the Guarded Suicidal Patient" and Chapter 7, "Patients at Acute and Chronic High Risk for Suicide: Crisis Management"). However, unlike physicians in other specialties, psychiatrists rarely encounter the death of a patient except by suicide. There are only two types of practicing psychiatrists—those who have experienced patient suicide and those who will.

Like doctors in all medical specialties, psychiatrists will have patients who die. This adverse outcome is inherent in the practice of medicine. A patient's death is a tragedy; however, it is not evidence, per se, of professional negligence. Nonetheless, malpractice suits against psychiatrists remain an occupational hazard. The treatment and safety management of suicidal patients can be anxiety-provoking and fatiguing. Some clinicians limit the number of patients at risk of suicide under their care. Others try to avoid treating suicidal patients altogether. Clinicians should realistically assess their ability to tolerate the uncertainty inherent in the treatment of suicidal patients.

Outpatients

A clinician's ability to exercise control over outpatients at risk for suicide, including those attending partial hospitalization programs, is limited. In outpatient settings, patient safety is usually managed by clinical interventions such as increasing the frequency of visits, strengthening the therapeutic alliance, providing or adjusting medication, and involving family or other concerned persons, if the patient permits. Voluntary or, if necessary, involuntary hospitalization remains an option for suicidal patients at high suicide risk who can no longer be safely treated as outpatients. Most suicidal patients at moderate suicide risk and some selected patients at high risk are treated as outpatients.

When to hospitalize a patient can be a challenging decision for the clinician. The decision is considerably more complicated when the need for hospitalization is clear but the patient refuses. The action that the clinician takes at this point is critical for the patient's treatment and for risk management. The clinician should not worry alone. Consultation is always an option.

The clinician, after systematic suicide risk assessment, determines that the patient requires hospitalization (see Chapter 7, "Patients at Acute and Chronic High Risk for Suicide: Crisis Management"). The risks and benefits of continuing outpatient treatment are weighed against the risks and benefits of hospitalization, and the assessment is shared with the patient. If the patient agrees, arrangements for immediate hospitalization are made. The patient must go *directly* to the hospital, accompanied by a responsible person. The patient should not stop to do errands, get clothing, have dinner, or make last-minute arrangements. A detour may provide the patient with the opportunity to attempt or to complete suicide. If the patient is driven to the hospital, a central safety-locking mechanism under the sole control of the driver, if available, may help prevent the patient from jumping out of the car. Suicidal individuals have jumped out of ambulances and other moving rescue vehicles, resulting in death or serious injuries. An additional passenger, preferably known to the patient, may be needed to accompany the patient. In some instances, clinicians have accompanied the patient to the hospital. The clinician, however, has no legal duty to assume physical custody of the patient (*Farwell v. Un* 1990).

If the patient rejects the clinician's recommendation for hospitalization, the matter is immediately addressed as a treatment issue. Because the need for hospitalization in such a case is acute, a prolonged inquiry into the patient's reasons for rejecting the recommendation for hospitalization is not feasible. Furthermore, the therapeutic alliance may be strained. Consultation and referral are options for the clinician to consider, if time and the patient's condition permit. It is this situation that challenges the professional and personal mettle of the clinician. The failure to involuntarily hospitalize a suicidal patient who subsequently attempts or completes suicide is a source of malpractice suits against outpatient clinicians. The uncompensated time required, inconvenience, disruption of the clinician's schedule, possibility of having to make a court appearance, and fear of a lawsuit by the patient may dissuade the clinician from initiating involuntary hospitalization. State commitment statutes grant clinicians immunity from liability when they use reasonable judgment, follow statutory commitment procedures, and act in good faith.

Documenting the suicide risk assessment and the rationale for involuntary hospitalization represents good clinical care as well as sound risk management. When involuntary hospitalization is sought, psychiatrists should leave it to the courts to resolve uncertainty about commitment. The clinician's proper focus is the patient's safety. For further discussion of involuntary hospitalization, see Chapter 7, "Patients at Acute and Chronic High Risk for Suicide: Crisis Management."

Split Treatment

Collaboration and communication between psychiatrist and psychotherapist in split-treatment settings are essential in assessing and managing the patient at risk for suicide. The essence of collaborative treatment is effective communication. The operative principle is, "We are in it together."

Psychiatrists and psychotherapists with split-treatment practices may not take the time or may not have the time available to adequately collaborate. For example, a psychiatrist who sees four patients for medication management every hour, 8 hours a day for 5 days a week, will treat 160 patients a week. Assuming the psychiatrist receives 20 patient telephone calls a day from a patient base of 500, the psychiatrist will receive 100 telephone calls a week, not including weekend calls. Extremely busy, high-volume medication management practices are common. How will the psychiatrist find the time to collaborate?

Collaboration takes time and effort. Communication is necessary to prevent the suicidal patient from falling between the cracks of split treatment (Gutheil and Simon 2003). Insurers, however, do not compensate clinicians for time spent in collaboration. Clinical responsibilities between psychiatrist and psychotherapist should be clearly demarcated to prevent role confusion and uncertainty, potentially increasing the patient's risk for suicide. Responsibility for patient emergencies should be clearly delineated. Adequate communication and collaboration between psychiatrist and psychotherapist is standard practice, especially for patients at risk for suicide.

Inpatients

In the managed care era, only the severely mentally ill are admitted to acute-care psychiatric facilities (Simon 1997). The purpose of hospitalization is crisis intervention, patient safety, and stabilization (Simon 1998). The criteria for voluntary admission often exceed the substantive standards required for involuntary hospitalization. Most patients are acutely suicidal, violent toward others, or both. Hospitalization is usually brief; the average stay in most short-term psychiatric facilities is between 3 and 5 days.

Patients who are potentially dangerous to themselves and others may be prematurely discharged (Simon 1998). The rapid admission, crisis management, and discharge of severely ill patients may not allow an overburdened staff enough time to thoroughly evaluate the new patient. Brief safety checks made by a succession of mental health personnel may not provide the time necessary to develop a relationship with the patient. Relying solely on a "promise" made or a no-harm contract signed by the patient saying he or she will not attempt suicide constitutes inadequate safety management (Simon 2004).

The level of supervision provided for patients at risk for suicide is determined after systematic assessment of suicide risk (Simon 1998). Suicide risk assessment is a process, not a single event, that gathers vital information to reduce the uncertainty surrounding patient treatment and safety management. Suicide prevention contracts should not be used in lieu of adequate suicide risk assessment (Garvey et al. 2009).

The treatment team has emerged as an important provider of care for psychiatric inpatients. Among its many advantages, the treatment team has "a thousand eyes" to focus on the safety supervision of suicidal patients. Nonetheless, the treatment team can develop blind spots when communication among team members is faulty, thus increasing the patient's risk for suicide. Inpatient suicides tend to occur shortly after admission, during staff shift changes, at meal times, when psychiatric residents finish their rotations, and after discharge (a few hours, days, or weeks later) (Qin and Nordentoft 2005). A newly admitted, severely mentally ill patient at significant risk for suicide who has not been treated by and is unknown to the clinical staff should be placed on suicide precautions according to the care needs of the patient. Patients who have made a serious suicide attempt just prior to admission will likely require one-to-one visual or arm's-length supervision. Nurses can exercise their discretion to place patients on suicide precautions or increase the precaution level if the psychiatrist cannot be reached or until the psychiatrist has an opportunity to call or to examine the patient. If suicide precautions are imposed by the nursing staff, the psychiatrist should assess the patient prior to discontinuance of the precaution and document the rationale for discontinuance or write an order to continue the precautions. Nurses cannot lower or discontinue suicide precautions.

Psychiatrists frequently receive phone calls from the nursing staff requesting a change or discontinuation of safety precautions regarding patients previously examined. Psychiatrists routinely make safety management decisions by phone, based on adequate on-the-spot suicide risk assessments performed by the clinical staff. A record of phone calls should be kept to prevent "he said, she said" controversies in case the phone call becomes a point of contention in a lawsuit.

Psychiatrists who admit inpatients during late-evening or early-morning hours need to evaluate the patient in a timely manner. Some psychiatric units allow psychiatrists up to 24 hours for the initial evaluation. This is unrealistic, given the severity of the illness at patient admission. Because of strict admission criteria, mostly patients at significant risk for suicide are admitted. The psychiatrist is placed in the difficult and legally exposed position of being responsible for the care of an unexamined suicidal patient who attempts or completes suicide.

In the context of the psychiatrist's initial evaluation of the newly admitted patient, "timeliness" is a purposely vague term. Much depends on the patient's psychiatric condition and level of suicide risk, as conveyed by the nursing staff. It is incumbent on the psychiatrist to ask as many questions of the clinical staff as necessary to obtain an adequate history upon which to base safety management of the patient. Until the patient can be seen, telephone checks with clinical staff may suffice. Patients who have made a serious suicide attempt leading to admission should be seen as soon as possible. The clinician may decide to see the patient at acute, high risk immediately after admission, if necessary.

Observation Levels

Systematic suicide risk assessment of the patient at admission informs the level of suicide precautions that must be taken. For example, does the patient require one-to-one, arm's-length, or close visual observation? Are safety checks every 15 or 30 minutes necessary, or is routine unit observation (usually every 30 minutes or hourly) sufficient? Psychiatrists should know the hospital's definition of *close observation*, which often varies among hospitals. It is usually easier to place a patient on suicide safety precautions than it is to reduce or discontinue precautions. Patients who are still on one-to-one or 15-minute safety observations should not be immediately discharged. Before being discharged, the patient should be observed for a period of time after suicide safety precautions are discontinued.

The usual practice is to initiate 15-minute checks on admission, with adjustment of the safety management as necessary. Automatic 15-minute checks, however, may not correspond to the patient's safety requirements. Patients can and do kill themselves between 15-minute checks. A patient who has made a near-lethal suicide attempt just prior to admission may require one-to-one supervision following the assessment.

High-volume admissions of acutely suicidal patients place a heavy burden on inpatient staffs. Limitation of services is a reality in the current managed care environment. Moreover, a patient determined to commit suicide can do it on one-to-one safety precautions. Busch et al. (2003), in a review of 76 inpatient suicides, found that 42 of these patients were on 15-minute suicide checks. In addition, 9% of patients were under one-to-one observation with a staff member at the time of suicide. They concluded that no specific suicide precautions are 100% effective.

When a patient at high risk for suicide is identified, one-to-one supervision may not be ordered, because insurance coverage for such services might not be available. Moreover, the hospital staff, stretched thin, may not be able to provide one-to-one patient supervision. The patient or family may be unable or unwilling to pay out-of-pocket for a "sitter." The psychiatrist or clinical staff should not place a high-risk patient in seclusion or restraint merely to obtain insurance coverage for one-to-one supervision. The use of seclusion and restraint is governed by strict clinical criteria and legal regulation. An acutely suicidal patient placed in seclusion and/or restraints requires one-to-one supervision. The temptation to obtain insurance coverage for such supervision by resorting to the questionable use of seclusion and restraint should be avoided.

Constant observation should be discontinued as soon as possible, consistent with the patient's safety requirement. The psychiatric unit is not a jail. Although safety is a primary concern, the decision to employ close observation must be balanced against the psychological distress it can cause the patient. For example, during close supervision, privacy in the performance of natural functions is lost. The patient cannot go to the bathroom or shower without the presence of an observer. Patients often experience intense embarrassment and humiliation that can increase hopelessness, depression, and suicide risk. Also, constant observation by a stranger is unnerving and intimidating, especially to a paranoid patient.

During periods of peak activity on the psychiatric unit, sufficient staff may not be available to provide one-to-one close observation. Without violating patient freedom-of-movement regulations, staff may "zone" the patient to an area in front of the nurses' station or to a specific location on the psychiatric unit where the patient can be kept under visual observation. Moreover, the clinical staff may not be able to provide time- and labor-intensive safety precautions at 5- or 10-minute intervals. Other patients are usually on suicide precautions. Five- or 10-minute safety checks and documentation may be overlooked, with potential liability consequences. If 5- to 10-minute checks are required, it may be better to place the patient on constant visual observation or on one-to-one arm's-length observation, monitored by either a staff member or a responsible, trained "sitter." Video monitoring can be inconsistent because of distractions of the staff on a busy unit.

After adequate initial assessment and observation, the newly admitted patient at risk for suicide who attends group meetings, socializes with other patients, and is visible on the unit usually has 15-minute checks discontinued. The patient is placed on standard ward supervision. In contrast, patients who are at high risk for suicide and are withdrawn and isolative may require one-to-one close observation. The persistently withdrawn, nonparticipating patient should be distinguished from a newly admitted patient who is initially isolated and withdrawn, but after a day or so feels more comfortable about being on a psychiatric unit. This adjustment occurs as the patient gradually establishes a relationship with staff members and peers. Observation levels must be flexible in order to accommodate patient needs. For example, a patient with melancholic depression may need closer supervision in the morning, when depressive symptoms are often worse.

Patients who have decided to commit suicide, however, may actually feel better or feign improvement. These patients usually "improve" suddenly, often dramatically, in contrast to patients whose genuine improvement is gradual but halting. In patients who have decided to commit suicide, core symptoms of psychiatric disorder (e.g., insomnia, anorexia, restlessness, and other symptoms of anxiety and depression) often persist. Distinguishing suicidal patients whose improvement is illusory from patients who are actually improving is one of the most difficult evaluations that psychiatrists must undertake. Psychiatrists' expectations that patients will improve while under their care can create a blind spot in safety assessment and management (see Chapter 6, "Sudden Improvement in Patients at High Risk for Suicide").

During peak periods of activity or shift changes on the unit, a suicidal patient may take advantage of the staff's distraction to attempt or commit suicide. The multidisciplinary team must be able to maintain consistent safety vigilance, even when it is stretched thin. If the psychiatric staff is understaffed or is overwhelmed by an influx of suicidal patients, temporary closure of the psychiatric unit to new admissions may be necessary. Just a few agitated, high-risk suicidal patients can fully occupy and quickly exhaust the clinical staff.

Imminent Suicide

Psychiatrists have difficulty gauging the imminence of suicide (Simon 2008). Imminence is not a psychiatric diagnosis. No risk factors identify imminence of suicide (see Chapter 11, "Imminent Suicide, Passive Suicidal Ideation, and Other Intractable Myths"). Suicide risk can vary by the minute, by the hour, or by the day. Patients are often considered to be at "imminent" risk for suicide when they are found to be hiding lethal instruments or when they are vocal about committing suicide at their first opportunity. Nonetheless, even suicidal individuals perched on bridges or with guns placed to their heads have been dissuaded from committing an intended lethal act. Some of the two dozen or so survivors who jumped from the Golden Gate Bridge changed their minds after they stepped off the bridge. Of 515 individuals who had been restrained from jumping, 94% were still alive many years later (Seiden 1978). It is imperative for the clinician to carefully assess, treat, and manage acute high-risk factors that are driving a suicide crisis rather than to attempt the impossible task of predicting when or whether a patient will attempt suicide (see Chapter 11, "Imminent Suicide, Passive Suicidal Ideation, and Other Intractable Myths").

Intensive Care Unit (Critical Care Unit)

The patient admitted to an intensive care unit (ICU) after a suicide attempt may be awaiting transfer to a psychiatric unit. In many hospitals, "sitters" are required to constantly attend the patient. A patient may seize an opportune moment to jump through an unsecured window in an ICU or medical/surgical unit or to walk off the ICU unit. Untrained "sitters" or family members rarely provide constant safety supervision. They often assume that the patient is compliant rather than devious in finding a way to commit suicide. They are reluctant to follow the suicidal patient into the bathroom. The patient may be able to commit suicide, usually by strangulation, while in the bathroom.

Medical/surgical units unintentionally provide many opportunities for the patient to commit suicide with unsecured equipment and other safety hazards. ICUs are not designed for the safety management of the psychiatric patient at risk for suicide. Transfer of the patient to the psychiatric unit should be a priority admission.

Seclusion and Restraint

The federal government's Center for Medicare & Medicaid Services (formerly the Health Care Financing Administration) (1999), The Joint Commission (formerly the Joint Commission on Accreditation of Healthcare Organizations [2001]), and most states have developed requirements designed to minimize or avoid the use of seclusion and restraint, wherever possible (Simon and Shuman 2007). Federal requirements may be superseded by more restrictive state laws. *Seclusion* is the involuntary confinement of a person alone in a room where the person is physically prevented from leaving, or the separation of the patient from others in a safe, contained, controlled environment. *Restraint* is the direct application of physical force to an individual, with or without the individual's permission, to restrict his or her freedom of movement. Physical force may involve human touch, mechanical devices, or a combination thereof. Use of these interventions presents an inherent risk to the patient's physical safety and well-being and, therefore, must be used only when there is a high risk that the patient may inflict harm to self or others. Statutory language may include the use of drugs in the definition of restraint (Simon and Shuman 2007). Seclusion and restraint should be used only as a last resort—and never for the convenience of staff. The indications and safety precautions for seclusion and restraint should be thoroughly documented. Seclusion and restraint should be used only when all other treatment and safety measures have failed. In such circumstances, the overarching therapeutic goal is to protect the patient's safety and dignity.

Qualified staff members may initiate seclusion or restraint for the safety and protection of the patient and staff; however, they must obtain an order from the licensed independent practitioner as soon as possible within 1 hour of initiation. Stringent requirements for face-to-face evaluation of the patient within 1 hour of initiation and for assessment, frequency of reassessment, monitoring, time-limited orders, notification of family members, discontinuation at the earliest possible opportunity, and debriefing with patient and staff members have been defined by the Center for Medicare & Medicaid Services and The Joint Commission.

More detailed indications and contraindications for seclusion and restraint can be found elsewhere and are beyond the scope of this chapter (American Psychiatric Association 1985). Seclusion and restraint may be necessary for the patient assessed at high risk for suicide in order to prevent self-harm. If the patient can be engaged by the staff shortly after admission, a nascent therapeutic alliance may develop. Appropriate medications given at therapeutic levels often stabilize the high-risk patient. If the suicidal patient is placed in seclusion and restraint, direct observation is required, according to regulatory and hospital policies. Seclusion rooms should have windows or audio-visual surveillance capability (Lieberman et al. 2004). Open-door seclusion is preferable when clinically appropriate.

Freedom of Movement

There must be a rational nexus between patient autonomy in the hospital setting and the patient's diagnosis, treatment, and safety needs. With patients at risk for suicide, standard safety precautions must be observed, such as removal of shoelaces, belts, sharps, glass products, and even pillowcases that can be used for suffocation. A thorough search for contraband on admission is standard procedure. Psychiatric units are usually fitted, at a minimum, with non-weight-bearing fixtures and shower curtain rods, break-away bed linens, paper washcloths, very short cords for electrical beds (properly insulated), cordless telephones or telephones with safety cords, jump-proof windows, barricade-proof doors, and closed-circuit video cameras. Plastic trash bags should not be used. The most common and available method of committing suicide by inpatients is strangulation, which is usually accomplished by a bed sheet hooked up to the patient's bed, door, or bathroom fixtures. Safe installation of plumbing pipes for toilets and use of solid ceilings are necessary to diminish the risk of hanging. The most dangerous place on the psychiatric unit is the patient's room, especially the bathroom.

Determining safety precautions is complicated by court directives that require highly disturbed patients to be treated by the least restrictive means (Simon 2000). In *Johnson v. United States* (1981), the court noted that an "open-door" policy creates a higher potential for danger. The court went on to say:

> Modern psychiatry has recognized the importance of making every effort to return a patient to an active and productive life. Thus, the patient is encouraged to develop his self-confidence by adjusting to the demands of everyday existence. Particularly because the prediction of danger is difficult, undue reliance on hospitalization might lead to prolonged incarceration of potentially useful members of society.

The tension between promoting individual freedom and preventing self-injury introduces an inherent uncertainty in the safety management of suicidal patients (Amchin et al. 1990). In malpractice suits, the individual facts of the case and the reasonableness of the staff's application of the open-door policy are determinative.

Policies and Procedures

Hospital policies and procedures require the patient to be evaluated by the psychiatrist within a specified period of time after admission. Departures from policies and procedures by the psychiatrist deserve a documented explanation. If the psychiatrist departs from the policies and procedures and the patient is harmed, a malpractice suit filed against the psychiatrist may be difficult to defend (*Eaglin v. Cook County Hospital* 1992). Official policies and procedures are consensus statements that often reflect the standard of care. However, they may propound "best practices" rather than the "ordinarily employed" standard care.

Departmental policy may require that a newly admitted patient remain on the psychiatric unit for a specified period of time, usually 24 hours. It is prudent not to issue off-ward privileges to new patients until their psychiatric evaluations are completed and safety needs determined. Emergency admissions of patients often occur late at night or in the early hours of the morning. Severely ill patients at high risk for suicide should be examined by the psychiatrist within a reasonable time after admission. The nursing staff has a duty to contact the psychiatrist in a timely manner after a patient is admitted.

In the managed care era, unaccompanied off-ward privileges or overnight passes for patients are a rarity. Staff-accompanied off-ward passes for in-hospital diagnostic procedures occur frequently. Depending on the urgency of the patient's medical problems and the level of assessed suicide risk, adequate supervision must be provided. In some cases, more than one staff member may be required to accompany the patient.

Newly admitted patients who smoke will often pressure the staff for a pass to go off-ward individually or with a smokers' group. The patient may reject a nicotine patch or inhaler. No off-ward pass should be issued unless the patient is cleared to have a pass after adequate assessment of suicide risk has been conducted and documented.

Premature Discharge

Patients leave the psychiatric unit against medical advice for a variety of reasons. Some smokers leave if they are not allowed to smoke on the unit. Patients with substance abuse disorders often sign out against medical advice, sometimes in the middle of the night. Informal (pure voluntary) and formal (conditional voluntary) admission policies determine whether the suicidal patient who demands to leave can be held for a period of evaluation. Purely voluntary patients cannot be held against their will. Only moral suasion can be used to encourage continued hospitalization. Just a few states continue to use informal admission procedures. In some hospitals, both psychiatric and addicted patients are admitted to the psychiatric unit. Patients admitted for substance detoxification may be informal admissions, whereas psychiatric patients on the same unit are formal admissions. Generally, substance-abusing patients without a comorbid psychiatric disorder cannot be held against their will, whereas substance-using patients with comorbid psychiatric disorders usually can be held against their will, if they are at risk for suicide.

The psychiatrist may not have had the opportunity to examine the patient and perform a suicide risk assessment before the patient decides to leave against medical advice. Reliance is placed on clinical staff members to conduct an adequate suicide risk assessment and to inform the psychiatrist of their evaluation. Conditional voluntary patients at significant risk for suicide can be held for a specified period of time for further evaluation. During the holding period, some patients withdraw their requests to leave and decide to stay. Other patients at low risk for suicide may be allowed to leave against medical advice or may be involuntarily hospitalized, if they remain at acute, high risk for suicide. The decision to release or retain a suicidal patient who signs out against medical advice depends on the assessed level of risk (Gerbasi and Simon 2003). Some patients at moderate to high suicide risk are treated as outpatients, especially when a working therapeutic alliance with an outpatient treater exists and other substantial protective factors are present.

Acutely suicidal patients seen in the emergency department who refuse hospitalization are usually confronted with making a choice between voluntary or involuntary hospitalization. Some patients opt for voluntary rather than involuntary hospitalization, only to seek discharge after a brief stay on the psychiatric unit. If the "revolving door" patient is a conditional (formal) voluntary admission, he or she can be held for further evaluation, as prescribed by state statute.

Suicide Warnings

The clinician has no legal duty to inform others that a patient is at risk for suicide (*Bellah v. Greenson* 1978). The *Tarasoff* duty to warn and protect endangered third parties, which exists in a number of jurisdictions, applies only if the threats of physical harm are directed toward others, not toward patients themselves (*Tarasoff v. Regents of the University of California* 1976). However, in *Gross v. Allen* (1994), a 1994 California appellate court case, the court held that if a patient has a history of dangerousness to self, the original caretaker is legally responsible for informing the new caretaker of this history. The court applied a *Tarasoff* analysis, extending the duty to warn and protect to threats of suicide.

Gross v. Allen does not appear to create a new duty for the psychiatrist in the safety management of patients at risk for suicide. Clinicians often communicate with new treaters after obtaining the patient's permission. Standard safety measures include communicating with significant others about the patient's condition, attempting to modify pathological interactions between the patient and family members, and mobilizing family support (e.g., removing lethal weapons, poisons, and drugs; administering and monitoring prescribed medications). Good clinical practice may require that significant others be apprised of the patient's risk of suicide or even to include them in the treatment, provided the patient agrees to such interventions. The patient, however, may not grant permission for disclosure. The clinician simply listening to others does not violate the patient's confidentiality. The patient should be informed of the telephone contact.

Principles of Medical Ethics With Annotations Especially Applicable to Psychiatry (American Psychiatric Association 2001) states, "Psychiatrists at times may find it necessary, in order to protect the patient or the community from imminent danger, to reveal confidential information disclosed by the patient" (Section 4, Annotation 8). Some states provide for statutory waiver of confidential information when a patient threatens self-harm (Simon 1992).

Significant Others

Cooperation and support of significant others in the patient's care are essential. Significant others include family members (spouse, mother, father, sibling, offspring, grandparent, other relatives) and nonfamily members (roommate, friend, fiancé, other) (Dervic et al. 2004). The family is often the patient's main support and protective factor against suicide. Postdischarge planning addresses the stability of the patient, the stability of the family, and the nature of the interaction between patient and family as important parts of the discharge risk-benefit assessment.

There are potential problems, however, with families providing patient supervision. First, the interaction between the patient and the family may be seriously impaired. Mentally ill patients frequently come from families that display significant psychological impairment. Moreover, some members of the patient's family may be more unstable than the patient. Family members may dissuade the patient from taking necessary medication because of their denial of the patient's mental illness. Disturbed families can become a risk factor for patient suicide. Educating the family about the patient's illness may help decrease destructive attitudes and behaviors that undermine the patient's stability and safety. Psychoeducation is important in postdischarge safety planning.

Family members are not trained to manage suicidal patients. Patients who are intent on killing themselves may find ingenious ways to attempt or commit suicide. Asking family members to keep a constant watch on the patient usually fails. Most family members will not follow the patient into the bathroom or be able to stay up all night to observe the patient. Moreover, family members find reasons to make exceptions to constant surveillance due to denial, fatigue, or the need to attend to other pressing matters. For example, one family who was told to keep the patient under constant watch allowed her to drive to church alone. She drove 30 miles to a bridge and jumped to her death.

There is an important role for the family, but it is not as a substitute for the constant safety management provided by trained mental health professionals on an inpatient psychiatric unit. Early discharge of an inpatient on the basis of reliance on family supervision can be precarious. If an outpatient at suicide risk requires constant 24-hour family supervision, then psychiatric hospitalization is indicated. Families, however, can be instructed to observe and report specific symptoms and behaviors displayed by the patient that often precede suicide attempts. Family support of the patient and feedback about the patient's thoughts and behaviors are appropriate, helpful roles. Family members who have a supportive relationship with the patient are often sensitive to important reportable changes in the patient's mental condition.

Therapeutic Risk Management

The fear of being sued can undermine patient safety management when clinically indicated interventions are compromised by a clinician's avoidant, defensive practices. The diffident, fearful clinician attempts to avoid the inherent uncertainties in the safety management of suicidal patients by adopting unduly defensive practices (Simon 1985, 1987). An affirmative, full commitment to the patient's care is lost. For example, a clinician who fails to involuntarily hospitalize a litigious, treatment-refusing patient at high risk for suicide, because he or she fears being sued, increases his or her liability exposure if the patient attempts or commits suicide.

Risk management is a reality of psychiatric practice, especially in the assessment and management of patients at risk for suicide. Risk management guidelines usually recommend *ideal* or *best* practices, whereas the actual standard of care is ordinary or reasonable care. Moreover, suicide cases are challenging, multifaceted, and nuanced, making it difficult to provide precise assessment and management guidelines.

Therapeutic risk management is patient-centered (Simon and Shuman 2009; see Chapter 13, "Therapeutic Risk Management of the Patient at Risk for Suicide: Clinical-Legal Dilemmas"). It supports the treatment process and the therapeutic alliance. At a minimum, it follows the fundamental ethical principle in medicine to "first do no harm." A working knowledge of the legal regulation of psychiatry enables the practitioner to more effectively manage psychiatric-legal issues that frequently arise with suicidal patients. Therapeutic risk management also provides the practitioner with a significant measure of comfort that supports the clinician's treatment role with patients at risk for suicide. Defensive practices that can undermine patient safety management are reduced.

Conclusion

The clinician's full commitment of time and effort to the care of the suicidal patient is the single most important factor in reducing the clinical uncertainties surrounding safety management. Uncertainty about clinical judgment calls is inevitable. Clinicians should assess their limits in coping with uncertainty and anxiety as well as the emotional and physical fatigue associated with the care of suicidal patients. Some clinicians limit the number of suicidal patents under their care or simply do not accept patients known to be at risk for suicide.

KEY CLINICAL CONCEPTS

- Effective treatment and safety management of the suicidal patient require the full commitment of time and effort from the clinician.

- Suicide risk assessment is a process, not an event. It is key to determining informed, ongoing treatment and safety management. It is performed on all patients at suicide risk.

- Suicide prevention contracts should not take the place of adequate suicide risk assessment. Reliance on suicide prevention contracts with new, unknown patients who are acutely ill is unwarranted. Suicide prevention contracts can create the illusion of safety where none exists.

- The entire treatment team participates in the supervision of the patient at suicide risk. The proper supervision of patients at risk for suicide in rapid-turnover inpatient settings cannot be the responsibility of only a few people.

- Families and other caretakers play an important part in safety management of the patient, especially when educated about their appropriate role. Most families, however, cannot provide constant supervision of the patient. If constant supervision is required, consider hospitalizing the patient or delaying discharge from the hospital until the patient is stabilized.

- Do not worry alone. Consultation is always an option.

References

Amchin J, Wettstein RM, Roth LH: Suicide, ethics, and the law, in Suicide Over the Life Cycle: Risk Factors, Assessment, and Treatment of Suicidal Patients. Edited by Blumenthal SJ, Kupfer DJ. Washington, DC, American Psychiatric Press, 1990, pp 637–663

American Psychiatric Association: The Psychiatric Uses of Seclusion and Restraint (Task Force Report No 22). Washington, DC, American Psychiatric Association, 1985

American Psychiatric Association: Principles of Medical Ethics With Annotations Especially Applicable to Psychiatry. Washington, DC, American Psychiatric Association, 2001

Bellah v Greenson, 81 Cal App 3d 614, 146, Cal Rptr 525 (1978)

Busch KA, Fawcett J, Jacobs DG: Clinical correlates of inpatient suicide. J Clin Psychiatry 64:14–19, 2003

Dervic K, Oquendo MA, Grunebaum MF, et al: Religious affiliation and suicide attempt. Am J Psychiatry 161:2303–2308, 2004

Eaglin v Cook County Hospital, 227 Ill App 3d 724, 592 NE2d 205 (1992)

Farwell v Un, 902 F2d 282 (4th Cir 1990)

Garvey KA, Penn JV, Campbell AL, et al: Contracting for safety with patients: clinical practice and forensic implications. J Am Acad Psychiatry Law 37:363–370, 2009

Gerbasi JB, Simon RI: When patients leave the hospital against medical advice: patient's rights and psychiatrists' duties. Harv Rev Psychiatry 11:333–334, 2003

Gross v Allen, 22 Cal App 4th 345, 27 Cal Rptr 2d 429 (1994)

Gutheil TG, Simon RI: Abandonment of patients in split treatment. Harv Rev Psychiatry 11:175–179, 2003

Health Care Financing Administration, 42 Code of Federal Regulation 482.13 (f)3 (II) (C) (1999)

Johnson v United States, 409 FSupp 1283 (MD Fla 1976), rev'd 576 F2d 606 (5th Cir 1978), cert denied, 451 U.S. 1019 (1981)

Joint Commission on Accreditation of Healthcare Organizations: Comprehensive Accreditation Manual for Behavioral Health Care: Restraint and Seclusion Standards for Behavioral Health. Chicago, IL, Joint Commission Accreditation of Healthcare Organizations, 2001, pp tx7.1.5–tx7.1.6

Lieberman DZ, Resnik HLP, Holder-Perkins V: Environmental risk factors in hospital suicide. Suicide Life Threat Behav 34:448–453, 2004

Qin P, Nordentoft M: Suicide risk in relation to psychiatric hospitalization. Arch Gen Psychiatry 62:427–432, 2005

Resnick PJ: Recognizing that the suicidal patient views you as an adversary. Curr Psychiatr 1:8, 2002

Seiden RH: Where are they now? A follow-up study of suicide attempters from the Golden Gate Bridge. Suicide Life Threat Behav 8:203–216, 1978

Simon RI: Coping strategies for the defensive psychiatrist. Med Law 4:551–561, 1985

Simon RI: A clinical philosophy for the (unduly) defensive psychiatrist. Psychiatr Ann 17:197–200, 1987

Simon RI: Clinical Psychiatry and the Law, 2nd Edition. Washington, DC, American Psychiatric Press, 1992

Simon RI: Discharging sicker, potentially violent psychiatric inpatients in the managed care era: standard of care and risk management. Psychiatr Ann 17:726–733, 1997

Simon RI: Psychiatrists' duties in discharging sicker and potentially violent inpatients in the managed care era. Psychiatr Serv 49:62–67, 1998

Simon RI: Taking the "sue" out of suicide: a forensic psychiatrist's perspective. Psychiatr Ann 30:399–407, 2000

Simon RI: Assessing and Managing Suicide Risk: Guidelines for Clinically Based Risk Management. Washington, DC, American Psychiatric Publishing, 2004

Simon RI: Imminent suicide: the illusion of short-term prediction. Suicide Life Threat Behav 38:517–522, 2008

Simon RI, Shuman DW: Clinical Manual of Psychiatry and Law. Washington, DC, American Psychiatric Publishing, 2007

Simon RI, Shuman DW: Therapeutic risk management of clinical-legal dilemmas: should it be a core competency? J Am Acad Psychiatry Law 37:156–161, 2009

Tarasoff v Regents of the University of California, 17 Cal3d 425, 551 P2d 334, 131 Cal Rptr 14 (1976)

CHAPTER 9

Gun Safety Management of Suicidal Patients

A Collaborative Approach

GUNS in the home are associated with a significant increase in suicide compared with homes without guns (Brent 2001). Regions with higher rates of home gun ownership have higher rates of suicide, after other factors associated with suicide have been controlled for (Barber 2005). In a study by Wintemute et al. (1999), the purchase of a handgun was associated with a significant increase in the risk of suicide by firearm and any other method. The increase in risk of a firearm suicide occurred within a week after purchase of a handgun, and the risk re-

Adapted with permission from Simon RI: "Gun Safety Management With Patients at Risk for Suicide." *Suicide and Life-Threatening Behavior* 37:518–526, 2007.

mained increased for at least 6 years. Within the first year of purchase, handguns accounted for 24.5% of all suicide deaths and 51.9% of deaths among women ages 21–33 years (Wintemute et al. 1999). In 2003, of the 31,484 suicides in the United States, 16,907 were by firearms (American Association of Suicidology 2006). Firearm suicide attempts end in death in approximately 85% of cases (Kellerman and Waecker 1998).

When lethal means of commiting suicide are less available, suicide rates decline by that method, and, often, overall suicide rates decline as well (Harvard School of Public Health 2010). In the United Kingdom, prior to 1958, domestic gas derived from coal contained 10%–20% carbon monoxide, a leading means of suicide. After 1958, natural gas, free of carbon dioxide, was introduced. A dramatic reduction in suicides occurred. Hawton (2002) estimated that 6,000–7,000 lives were saved by the switch to natural gas. Means reduction saves lives by decreasing the lethality of suicide attempts, not the intent to commit suicide. Gun safety management is a critical clinical intervention in reducing patient suicides.

The method of storage and the number of guns in the home influence suicide risk. The risk of suicide associated with guns in the home is higher for handguns than for long guns, for unlocked guns than for locked guns, and for loaded guns than for unloaded guns (Brent 2001). Total suicide rates have a statistical association to household gun prevalence (Markush and Bartolucci 1984). Persons with guns at home were more likely to have died from a firearm suicide than by suicide from a different method (Dahlberg et al. 2004).

Most patients at moderate risk for suicide are treated as outpatients (Simon 2004). Carefully selected patients assessed to be at high risk for suicide also may be treated as outpatients. However, most psychiatric patients at high risk for suicide are hospitalized. Patients evaluated in the emergency department are often at moderate to high risk for suicide. Some patients have guns stored at home or elsewhere (e.g., cars, workplace, or with others). Patients at risk for suicide must be asked about the availability and accessibility of guns.

Impulsivity and guns are a lethal mixture. In a study by Simon et al. (2001), suicide attempters ages 15–34 years were asked how much time they had spent between the decision to complete suicide and the attempt. Overall, 5% reported spending 1 second, and 24% stated that they had spent less than 5 minutes. Suicide rehearsal with a gun reinforces the belief that a firearm suicide is quick and easy. The gun is placed to the

TABLE 9–1.	Principles of gun safety management with patients at risk for suicide

- Inquire about guns at home or located outside the home (e.g., car, office, elsewhere). Also, inquire if patient intends to obtain or purchase a gun.
- Designate a willing, responsible person to remove and safely secure guns and ammunition outside the home, at a location unknown to the patient.
- Have direct contact with or receive a phone call from the designated person, confirming that guns and ammunition are properly removed from the home or from outside the home and safely secured according to the prearranged gun safety management plan. E-mail should not be used to communicate.
- Do not discharge inpatients or emergency department patients assessed as at risk for suicide until guns and ammunition are properly removed and secured.[a]

[a]For outpatients, decide on case-by-case basis.

head or in the mouth and death is only a trigger-click away. It takes less time to reach for a loaded gun than most other methods of suicide (e.g., overdose, hanging, carbon monoxide). Within a few minutes, the acute, time-limited impulse to commit suicide may pass.

Principles of Gun Safety Management

Gun safety management of patients at risk for suicide can be a complex, difficult challenge. Total prevention of suicide by any method is an impossible task. Nonetheless, practitioners must be proficient in providing competent clinical gun safety management (see Table 9–1).

Every psychiatric disorder except mental retardation is associated with an increased risk of suicide (Harris and Barraclough 1997; see Chapter 5, "Psychiatric Disorders and Suicide Risk"). Should psychiatric patients be routinely asked if they have guns at home? If the answer is affirmative, should the patient be informed of research that demonstrates an increased risk of suicide when guns are in the home?

Should the clinician advise psychiatric patients, regardless of suicide risk, to have guns removed from the home? Should only patients at current low risk for suicide but with a family history of suicide receive such a recommendation? In answering these questions, the decision to inform and intervene can only be determined by reasoned clinical judgment and discretion applied case by case. Asking patients who are not at current risk for suicide about guns in the home may unduly alarm the patient and disrupt a fledgling treatment. Patients at risk for suicide, however, require active implementation of a clinical gun safety management plan.

Gun safety management is first and foremost a treatment issue, but the clinician must do more if the patient is at risk for suicide (American Psychiatric Association 2003). Suicidal patients must be asked if they have access to guns. Some patients will volunteer that they have guns at home. Other patients will deny that there are guns at home, even though guns are easily accessible elsewhere. Thus, it is necessary to ask the patient, "Do you have guns at home or at any other place?" "Can you get one easily?" Additionally, the patient should be asked, "Do you intend to obtain or purchase a gun?" In one study, it was reported that in the first week following the purchase of a handgun, suicide by firearms among purchasers was 57 times higher than the adjusted rate for the general population (Wintemute et al. 1999).

Patients who have a gun at home usually have more than one gun. Guns that are described as locked up and safely stored can still be accessible, for example, if the patient has a duplicate key or is able to break into the place where the guns are stored. The clinician should not rely on "no-harm contracts" given orally or in writing by the patient as part of gun safety management; no evidence exists that such suicide prevention contracts reduce or eliminate suicide risk (Simon 2004; Stanford et al. 1994).

All handguns and long guns must be removed, along with ammunition, and stored in a place not accessible to the patient. But who will do it? The patient may want to give the guns to a family member or other persons for safekeeping. This option is risky because it places the patient in direct contact with guns. In some instances, patients have brought guns to the clinician for safekeeping. The risk to the clinician is obvious. The danger of harm persists when the patient requests that the guns held by the clinician be returned. If the clinician disagrees, a counter-therapeutic power struggle may develop that undermines the treatment. It is not the responsibility of the clinician to provide safe storage of patients' firearms.

In an optimal situation, the patient at risk for suicide acknowledges that guns are at home and agrees to have the guns removed by a designated, responsible person, usually a family member, partner, or neighbor. The treatment boundaries are thus readjusted to accommodate the designated person. The designated individual must be able to remove the gun(s) without self-injury and, if unable to do so, to contact a capable person or the police to perform the task. The designated person may require competent assistance in disarming the gun(s). Many individuals do not know how to handle firearms or are fearful when around guns.

By a prearranged plan, the designated individual will report back to the clinician that all guns have been removed from the home or from outside the home and safely secured, so that the guns and ammunition cannot be found by the patient. As tragic events demonstrate, simply hiding guns does not suffice. Patients intent on completing suicide find ingenious ways to obtain guns that are supposedly secured in the home. The patient at risk for suicide may be able to unlock guns with trigger locks or may have a duplicate key for guns stored in lock boxes or gun safes. He or she may have a combination number written down somewhere or may know some other way of defeating formal locking devices to access guns. The negotiations among the clinician, the patient, and the designated individual must be fully documented.

The clinician cannot rely on a task-specific therapeutic alliance with the person designated to implement the gun safety plan, unless that individual is in conjoint treatment with the patient at risk for suicide. The clinician's task is to determine whether the designated person understands the gun safety plan and is responsible enough to carry it out; that determination is a clinical judgment call. All the clinician can do is to trust his or her assessment and *verify* it by arranging a return call from the designated person to confirm that the safety plan has been executed in the agreed upon manner. Some might prefer to verify, then trust.

Instructions on gun safety management must be kept as simple and straightforward as possible. Discussion of this subject can often cause the patient's family or partner to be frightened and easily confused. In such cases, asking the designated person to remove the firing pin of a gun or securing the gun in a combination locking safe, with the combination reset, may overwhelm the designated person and scuttle the safety plan.

A meeting with the patient, the designated responsible person, and the clinician should be arranged, if possible. All participants should be encouraged to ask and answer questions freely. A collaborative, team approach helps to preserve the therapeutic alliance and gives the clinician the opportunity to meet the designated person. It should be explained that guns in the home increase the risk of suicide. The designated person should be instructed to go directly home, immediately remove the guns and ammunition from the home, and transfer the guns to safe storage outside the home, at a location unknown to the patient. Loaded guns must be disarmed. The designated person agrees to call back once the task is performed expeditiously. All other daily tasks and activities should be deferred. If no callback is received or is not received in a prearranged, timely manner, the patient's gun safety plan is no longer viable. Limitations exist on the ability of the clinician to ensure that the patient and designated person will comply with a gun safety management plan.

In a study by Brent et al. (2000), the parents of 106 adolescents with major depression participated in a randomized psychotherapy clinical trial. Those parents who answered "yes" to having guns at home were urged to remove them after being informed of the suicide risk. Only 27% removed guns by the end of the acute trial. The authors concluded that families of depressed adolescents were noncompliant with recommendations to remove guns despite being compliant with other aspects of treatment. Although a small-scale study by Kruesi et al. (1999) demonstrated that parental education on injury prevention limited access to firearms, larger scale studies by Grossman et al. (2000) and Sidman et al. (2005), showed that a safety counseling session or a multifaceted community education campaign to promote safe firearm storage did not lead to statistically significant changes in gun storage practices. These studies underscore the importance of a callback from the designated person to confirm implementation of the agreed-upon gun safety management plan.

In a situation involving a patient at risk for suicide, time and circumstances may not allow for a meeting with a person designated to remove guns from a patient's home. In that case, phone contact with the designated person familiar with the situation should be made, preferably with the patient present, in which it is explained that the gun(s) and ammunition must be removed immediately and stored separately in a safe place *outside* the home, as described earlier in this chapter. A "cold call" should be avoided, if possible. Such calls can alarm an un-suspecting recipient, making it difficult for that person to assimilate the clinician's instructions and to ask questions. It is preferable to have the patient call the designated person first. Telephone contact with a des-ignated person is less than optimal, but it may be the only pragmatic alternative. In any event, the clinician must be satisfied that the gun safety management plan is clearly understood, either by direct contact or by telephone. E-mail contact with designated persons is insufficient; an actual conversation is necessary so that the clinician may discern nuances and ambiguities and avoid misunderstandings. Family mem-bers may hide a gun in a place that they think is safe, but it may be easily found by the patient who is determined to attempt suicide. It is a clinical axiom that there is no safe gun storage at a suicidal patient's home. Again, the gun safety plan should be carefully documented.

Eventually, the patient may ask that the guns be returned. When the therapeutic alliance with the patient is present and cooperation by the designated third-party exists, an informed decision to return the guns to the patient is made jointly by the clinician, the patient, and the des-ignated person. In the absence of such collaboration, the clinician may have little or no control over the premature release of gun(s) to the pa-tient. The gun safety plan, at its inception, should include a discussion about the clinical criteria that will be considered in the decision to re-turn a gun(s) to a patient.

Application of Gun Safety Management Principles

The application of gun safety management principles varies across treatment settings, specific clinical situations, and the safety require-ments of patients at risk for suicide.

Outpatients

The opportunities for gun safety management of suicidal patients in outpatient settings are limited. Much depends on whether the patient is a new or an established patient, a therapeutic alliance with the patient is present or absent, supportive relationships with responsible individuals are available, and other protective factors. Systematic suicide assessments that consider both risk and protective factors guide the clinician's decision (Simon 2006).

Asking an outpatient to stay in the waiting area while guns are being removed from the home and secured elsewhere may be workable on a case-by-case basis. It may, however, be unnecessary, impractical, and counter-therapeutic. Patients are free to leave an outpatient setting at any time. Clinicians cannot restrict an outpatient's freedom of movement unless the patient is petitioned for involuntary hospitalization. If it is necessary to ask the patient to wait until guns are removed from the home, hospitalization should be considered. The patient at risk for suicide who lives alone and is isolated from others may not be able to identify a designated person for gun removal. Hospitalization may be required while the gun(s) are removed by other means.

Even with the most cooperative patient, the clinician cannot provide suicide-proof gun safety management. There are too many suicide risk variables beyond the clinician's control. For example, between sessions, a stable therapeutic alliance may be undermined by an unexpected surge in the severity of the patient's illness or by unanticipated traumatic events. Then again, individuals entrusted with the responsibility for removing and securing guns may fail to follow the safety plan. If a patient who is assessed at moderate to high risk of suicide refuses to cooperate with the clinician in securing guns at home, then voluntary or, if necessary, involuntary hospitalization may be required for the patient's safety. Patients intent on completing suicide often regard the clinician as their enemy (Resnick 2002). Hidden guns may not be disclosed. However, all the clinician can do is implement a reasonable gun safety management plan in order to reduce the risk of a firearm suicide.

A patient at risk for suicide may refuse authorization for the clinician to speak with others for the purpose of securing guns. The patient may not want family members or a partner to know that he or she is suicidal and has guns hidden at home. In that case, the clinician must determine whether the situation is an emergency necessitating a breach of confidentiality. The *Principles of Medical Ethics With Annotations Especially Applicable to Psychiatry* (American Psychiatric Association 2001) states, "A psychiatrist at times may find it necessary, in order to protect the patient or community from imminent danger, to reveal confidential information disclosed by the patient" (Section 4, Annotation 8). Mental health clinicians in other disciplines should consult their professional organization guidelines regarding how to manage the tension between maintaining patient confidentiality versus disclosure in emergency situations.

Under the Health Insurance Portability and Accountability Act of 1996 (HIPAA), it is permissible for covered providers to disclose information in emergencies without the patient's authorization, within certain guidelines (Vanderpool 2002). In an emergency, consent for treatment is also implied (Simon and Goetz 1999). Federal and state statutes and courts define *medical emergency* along a spectrum from narrow to expansive (Currier et al. 2002).

When confronted with a choice between maintaining patient confidentiality and disclosing information critical to the suicidal patient's safety, the clinician should err on the side of life and disclose. Moreover, it is better to take a chance on being sued for breach of confidentiality than to lose a patient to suicide.

Inpatients

Many patients admitted to a psychiatric unit have severe psychiatric disorders and are at high suicide risk. The hospital length of stay is very brief, usually 5 or 6 days, or less. Inpatients are often discharged at some level of reduced suicide risk. Inpatient treatment is designed to stabilize the patient. Postdischarge planning addresses the patient's need for further treatment and safety management.

The inpatient gun safety management team includes the psychiatrist, patient, clinical staff, and a designated responsible person (e.g., family member, partner, other). To prevent miscommunications that can develop when the psychiatrist must respond to multiple family members, the designated person should be the main contact person throughout the patient's hospitalization.

The clinical team, as part of the initial screening, must ask the patient if there are guns at home or easily accessible elsewhere. The patient may admit to possessing guns and disclose their location, he or she may only partially disclose the location of guns at home, or he or she may deny accessibility to guns. With the patient's written permission, a person who lives with the patient should also be asked to verify the presence and location of guns disclosed by the patient as well as the possible possession and location of other firearms. The psychiatrist should then meet with the designated responsible person in the presence of the patient, given that the patient's cooperation is essential to the gun safety management. The gun safety plan should then be explained, agreed on, and documented.

Determining a designated person's ability to competently execute the gun removal plan can be more problematic in situations involving an inpatient. The mental stability of the designated person may be difficult to determine by phone. Some family members or partners may be more mentally disordered than the patient. If the patient does not grant permission to contact family members or partners in order to implement a gun safety plan, the patient's discharge should be delayed while other treatment and safety options are pursued.

An inpatient at risk for suicide who lives alone and is isolated from others may have guns at home but no person to designate for gun removal. Upon reflection, the patient may be able to think of someone who could act as a designated person. If no family or friend can be found, the patient should be encouraged to call the local police precinct to have the guns impounded. The patient's refusal to cooperate is a contraindication for discharge until the gun safety issue is resolved. The staff will need to provide the police with a legitimate reason to enter the patient's home. The police option will require the active participation of the staff, who will provide the patient's house key and inform the police of the location of the guns. The police will call back to confirm that the guns were removed. The patient must be told that the police may not return the guns, depending on the jurisdiction. Patients who are gun enthusiasts, sportsmen, and hunters, will not want their guns impounded by the police, prompting them to find another option for gun removal. Legislative remedies may also be helpful. State laws should be consulted to determine limitations or facilitation of the clinician's gun safety management plan (Norris et al. 2006).

Gun safety management requires that before the patient is discharged, the guns at home or stored elsewhere must continue to be secured. Recently discharged psychiatric patients are at increased risk of suicide, especially within the week following discharge (Currier et al. 2002). If guns are kept with the patient's friends or acquaintances, they must be informed explicitly not to allow the patient to retrieve the guns. It is critical that the responsible party call the psychiatrist or clinical staff to verify that the gun(s) is safely secured before the patient is discharged. The callback allows the clinician to determine whether the gun removal plan was properly performed (e.g., where the guns are stored). If no call is received from the responsible party within the agreed upon time, the patient's discharge should be delayed until the guns can be secured. A follow-up call by the psychiatrist or clinical staff may be made to the designated person responsible for removing the guns. The clinical staff, however, cannot be expected to track down persons who fail to call back as previously agreed.

Delays in patient discharges can be lessened when the safety management plan is activated on the first day of admission. Trying to remove guns and receiving a verification call at the last minute may lead to a delay in discharge, patient regression, and the denial of insurance coverage for additional unauthorized hospital days. Worse, it may abort the safety plan, if the patient insists on discharge and the responsible person cannot be located to secure the firearms. Any delays or complications regarding gun removal must halt the patient's discharge until the problems are resolved.

A gun removal plan for an inpatient may fail for a variety of reasons. The person responsible for securing guns may give an affirmative callback that the guns have been moved according to plan but could then delay in securing the guns. The designated person may become distracted or change his or her mind about gun safety, disbelieving that the patient would attempt suicide based on the patient's disavowal of suicide. Often, family, partners, or a friend's denial of the patient's suicide intent is a major factor in nonadherence to safe gun removal from the home. Another possibility is that the patient's or family member's car is not checked for guns. The designated person may or may not know that there is a gun at the patient's place of employment. Because of ambivalence, exhaustion, or frustration with a seriously ill suicidal patient, family members may not diligently follow the agreed-upon plan and may carelessly store guns where the patient can find them. Moreover, the patient may undermine a discharge gun safety plan by withholding information about the existence of other guns. Some family members lie about removal of guns in order to have the patient discharged. The clinician is not a detective. Affirmation of adherence to the gun safety plan by a designated person is, by necessity, taken at face value.

Despite the many potential pitfalls, clinicians must perform adequate suicide risk assessments and implement a gun safety plan prior to discharge. Gun safety management is an essential component in the patient's postdischarge treatment plan. As discussed in this chapter, the outpatient clinician must decide when or if it is safe to return guns to the patient. A continuation of the gun safety management plan is an integral part of a careful "hand off" of the patient from inpatient to outpatient treatment.

Emergency Patients

Patients at high risk for suicide by firearms are routinely evaluated in the emergency department. Every psychiatric patient admitted to the emergency department *must* be asked about a suicide plan by firearms, the accessibility of firearms, or the intent to obtain firearms. In some instances, suicidal patients have brought guns into the emergency department. Some emergency departments have a metal detection security system for the protection of the staff and patients. As noted in the study by Wintemute et al. (1999), the recent purchase of a handgun by a suicidal patient is an indicator of high risk, especially in women ages 21–33 years. When a suicidal patient is admitted to the emergency department, the patient is initially examined by a physician. Once the patient is medically cleared, a crisis counselor usually evaluates the patient. The task of the crisis counselor is to quickly gather as much information as possible to make an appropriate disposition. If the patient has been previously admitted to the emergency department or the inpatient unit, the patient's records should be requested and reviewed. Electronic records are often available for immediate review. The clinician should attempt to contact the treating therapists, if the patient is in current treatment. Because patients are often admitted late at night or in the early morning hours, information gathering may be limited. Most patients will provide names and phone numbers for the crisis counselor to contact. The patient's history, including the presence and location of guns in the home, should be verified with the contact person. The emergency department is a prime venue for suicide prevention, given the sheer number of patients at risk for suicide who come through its doors.

When a patient at risk for suicide in the emergency department is admitted to an inpatient unit, gun safety management is transferred to the inpatient clinical staff. If it is determined that the patient's risk of suicide can be managed as an outpatient and that guns are accessible at home, the team safety plan described earlier in this chapter should be implemented and documented. Patients at risk for suicide who are referred for outpatient treatment the next day or next few days must have guns removed from the home and safely secured before discharge from the emergency department. If a responsible party is not available to secure the guns or if a reasonable doubt exists that the gun safety plan can be effectively implemented, the patient should be admitted to the inpatient unit for further evaluation and treatment. Merely asking and documenting, "No SI, HI, or CFS" (no suicidal ideation, homicidal ideation, or contracts for safety) and sending the patient home is unacceptable. Systematic suicide risk assessment that informs treatment and safety management is required (Simon 2006).

If the patient requires constant 24-hour surveillance following discharge from the emergency department, he or she should be admitted to the inpatient unit. The patient's family or partner should not be burdened with the impossible task of providing constant one-to-one supervision of the patient. Exceptions to constant supervision are invariably made by family members. For example, it is rare that the patient will be followed into a bathroom. Distractions also occur as a result of the activities of daily living. Family members assume that the patient wants help. They deny or downplay that the patient is determined to die and is looking for a gun or other means to complete suicide.

The safety management plan proposed here is only one method of reducing gun suicides. Other viable approaches to gun safety management will depend on the clinician's training, clinical experience, and the unique treatment and safety management needs of the individual patient. Whatever method of gun safety management is adopted, it should employ a team approach with prearranged callback verification from the responsible, designated person to confirm that the patient's guns have been disarmed and removed from the home and are safely secured. The essence of gun safety management is verification.

Conclusion

Guns in the home are associated with a significant increase in suicide. All patients at risk for suicide must be asked if guns are available at home or easily accessible elsewhere, or if they have intent to buy or purchase a gun. Gun safety management requires a collaborative team approach including the clinician, patient, and designated person responsible for removing guns from the home. A call-back to the clinician from the designated person is required confirming that guns have been removed and secured according to plan. The principle of gun safety management applies to outpatients, inpatients, and emergency patients, although its implementation varies according to the clinical setting.

KEY CLINICAL CONCEPTS

- The essence of gun safety management is verification.

- Gun safety management requires a collaborative, team approach.

- Guns in the home are associated with a significant increase in suicide compared with homes without guns.

- Impulsivity and guns are a lethal combination. The time between decision and suicide attempt is often a matter of a few seconds or minutes.

- The purchase of a handgun is associated with a significant increase in the risk of suicide within a week of purchase.

References

American Association of Suicidology: U.S.A. Suicide: 2003 official final data. 2006. Available at: http://dhhs.nv.gov/Suicide/DOCS/StatisticsResearch/AllStateSuicideRankings/2003%20Final%20Data.pdf. Accessed January 26, 2010.

American Foundation for Suicide Prevention: Firearms and suicide. 2010. Available at: http://www.afsp.org/index.cfm?fuseaction=home.viewPage&page_id=0ABB1629-08A0-ACE7-DEBF9EAE00C45352. Accessed January 26, 2010.

American Psychiatric Association: Principles of Medical Ethics With Annotations Especially Applicable to Psychiatry. Washington, DC, American Psychiatric Association, 2001, Section 4, Annotation 8

American Psychiatric Association: Practice guidelines for the assessment and treatment of patients with suicidal behaviors. Am J Psychiatry 160 (suppl 11):1–60, 2003

Barber CW: Fatal connection: the link between guns and suicide. Advancing Suicide Prevention 1:25–26, 2005

Brent DA: Firearms and suicide. Ann N Y Acad Sci 932:225–240, 2001

Brent D, Baugher M, Birmaher B, et al: Compliance with recommendations to remove firearms in families participating in a clinical trial for adolescent depression. J Am Acad Child Adolesc Psychiatry 39:1226–1228, 2000

Currier GW, Allen MH, Serper MR, et al: Medical, psychiatric, and cognitive assessment in the psychiatric emergency service, in Emergency Psychiatry. Edited by Allen MH (Review of Psychiatry Series, Vol 21; Oldham JM and Riba MB, series eds). Washington, DC, American Psychiatric Publishing, 2002, pp 35–74

Dahlberg LL, Ideda RM, Kresnow M: Guns in the home and risk of violent death in the home: findings from a national study. Am J Epidemiol 160:929–936, 2004

Grossman DC, Cummings P, Koepsell TD, et al: Firearm safety counseling in primary care pediatrics: a randomized controlled trial. Pediatrics 106:22–26, 2000

Harris CE, Barraclough B: Suicide as an outcome for mental disorders. Br J Psychiatry 170:205–228, 1997

Harvard School of Public Health: Means matter: means reduction saves lives. 2010. Available at: http://www.hsph.harvard.edu/means-matter/means-matter/saves-lives/index.html. Accessed January 27, 2010.

Hawton K: United Kingdom legislation on pack sizes of analgesics: background, rationale and effects on suicide and deliberate self-harm. Suicide Life Threat Behav 32:223–229, 2002

Kruesi MJ, Grossman J, Pennington JM, et al: Suicide and violence prevention: parent education in the emergency department. J Am Acad Child Adolesc Psychiatry 38:250–255, 1999

Kellerman AL, Waecker LE: Preventing firearm injuries. Ann Emerg Med 33:77–79, 1998

Markush RE, Bartolucci AA: Firearms and suicide in the United States. Am J Public Health 2:123–127, 1984

Norris DM, Price M, Gutheil TG, et al: Firearm laws, patients, and the roles of psychiatrists. Am J Psychiatry 163:1392–1396, 2006

Resnick PJ: Recognizing that the suicidal patient views you as an adversary. Curr Psychiatr 1:8, 2002

Sidman EA, Grossman DC, Koepsell TD, et al: Evaluation of a community-based handgun safe-storage campaign. Pediatrics 115:654–661, 2005

Simon OR, Swann AC, Powell KE, et al: Characteristics of impulsive suicide attempts and attempters. Suicide Life Threat Behav 32 (suppl 1):49–59, 2001

Simon RI: Assessing and Managing Suicide Risk: Guidelines for Clinically Based Risk Management. Washington, DC, American Psychiatric Publishing, 2004

Simon RI: Suicide risk: assessing the unpredictable, in The American Psychiatric Publishing Textbook of Suicide Assessment and Management. Edited by Simon RI, Hales RE. Washington, DC, American Psychiatric Publishing, 2006, pp 1–32

Simon RI, Goetz S: Forensic issues in the psychiatric emergency department. Psychiatr Clin North Am 22:851–864, 1999

Stanford EJ, Goetz RR, Bloom JD: The no harm contract in the emergency assessment of suicide risk. J Clin Psychiatry 55:344–348, 1994

Vanderpool D: HIPAA privacy rule: an update for psychiatrists. Psychiatric Practice and Managed Care 8:5–12, 2002

Wintemute GJ, Parham CA, Beaumont JJ, et al: Mortality among recent purchasers of handguns. N Engl J Med 341:1583–1589, 1999

CHAPTER 10

Suicide Risk Assessment Forms

Clinician Beware

SUICIDE risk assessment is a core competency that informs patient treatment and management (Scheiber et al. 2003). It is a process of analysis and synthesis that identifies, prioritizes, and integrates acute and chronic risk and protective factors into an overall assessment of the patient's suicide risk.

Psychiatrists assess suicidal patients who present life-threatening emergencies. Unlike other physicians, psychiatrists do not have laboratory tests and sophisticated diagnostic instruments to assess patients at risk for suicide. For example, when evaluating an emergency cardiac patient, the physician orders a number of diagnostic tests and procedures such as electrocardiography, serial enzymes, imaging, and catheteriza-

Adapted from Simon RI: "Suicide Risk Assessment: Form Over Substance?" *Journal of American Academy of Psychiatry and Law* 37:290–293, 2009. © American Academy of Psychiatry and the Law. Reprinted with permission.

tion to provide clinical data that are analyzed and synthesized into an overall treatment and management plan. For the suicidal patient, the psychiatrist's diagnostic instrument is systematic suicide risk assessment.

Patients at risk for suicide can evoke a variety of troubling emotions in the clinician that cause anxiety, sleep disturbances, and distraction. Countertransference anger, hate, and a reaction formation of solicitude toward the suicidal patient can threaten the clinician's ability to assess and treat the patient competently (Gabbard and Allison 2006). A patient's suicide is devastating, arousing powerful feelings of grief, guilt, betrayal, anger, depression, and loss of clinical confidence (Gitlin 2006). Charles and Kennedy (1985) eloquently described the serious personal and professional consequences of a lawsuit following a patient's suicide. Thus, clinicians may resort to use of suicide risk assessment forms as a risk management technique, in the illusory belief that a form can provide a defense or deterrence against a malpractice suit. Unfortunately, assessment forms merely cast a spell of reassurance, often masquerading as competent clinical assessment and judgment. The clinician is left with the false notion that further clinical assessment of suicide risk is unnecessary, paradoxically exposing the clinician to increased liability risk.

In suicide malpractice cases, plaintiffs' attorneys will closely scrutinize a suicide risk assessment form. Invariably, the patient who attempts or completes suicide has displayed risk factors not included on the form. The attorney's expert will then testify that, instead of relying on an assessment form, had the clinician performed a competent suicide risk assessment, the patient's increased suicide risk would have become apparent.

Fantasy Forms

Suicide risk assessment forms (hereafter referred to as "form[s]") are endemic. They are created by mental health professionals with a wide variety of training and experience. Of the plethora of current forms in existence, no two are alike. Many forms soon disappear, often after a patient's suicide, only to be replaced by another short half-life form. Some forms become institutionalized, achieving a long life of their own, despite multiple occurrences of suicides.

Forms do not possess psychometric properties; that is, they are not tested for reliability and validity. Some forms are designed to be scored and totaled to reach a numerical overall assessment of suicide risk. The resulting score creates a fiction of added accuracy, further misleading the clinician. Suicide risk assessment cannot be reduced to a number.

Forms are favored by clinicians who treat patients in inpatient settings where rapid patient turnover and short lengths of stay occur. Seriously ill inpatients at high risk for suicide often evoke anxiety among the clinical staff, who then place their confidence in checked-off forms. Similarly, in busy outpatient medication management practices, assessment forms that can be quickly filled out within a brief visit are preferred. Checklists are frequently used in emergency departments, usually requiring an accompanying documented narrative that describes the suicide risk assessment process. It is much easier to check-off a form than to conduct a thorough suicide risk assessment. Unfortunately, there are no shortcuts or quick fixes for conducting a competent suicide risk assessment.

Another fundamental flaw of suicide risk forms is the absence of a process of analysis and synthesis. The clinician is not required to identify, prioritize, and integrate risk and protective factors into an *overall* assessment of the patient's suicide risk. Form trumps substance.

Another basic limitation found on many forms is their failure to determine the presence or absence of protective factors. Protective factors require the same thorough assessment as do risk factors. A clinical assessment that considers only risk factors is incomplete and flawed.

Forms often contain impressionistic risk factors that the creator(s) erroneously believes are reliable indicators of suicide risk. Some forms seem to be created out of thin air. For example, "emotional pain," "insight," and "self-hate," which may be applicable to a specific patient, are not evidence-based, *general* suicide risk factors. Some forms contain cartoon-like facial expressions depicting a spectrum of mood from happy to profoundly depressed.

Forms often display a paucity of evidence-based suicide risk and protective factors. For example, psychiatric diagnosis, an important suicide risk factor, is often omitted. Other important evidence-based risk factors are glaringly absent, such as psychosis; melancholia; eating disorders; hopelessness; anxiety/agitation; insomnia; panic; impulsivity; anhedonia; substance abuse; recent interpersonal loss; comorbidity; and firearms in the home. In contrast, so-called shotgun forms include a bewildering list of suicide risk factors, some relevant, many not, that produce eye-glazing, robotic check-offs denoting their presence or absence. No explanatory assessment narrative accompanies the checklist.

Patient self-assessment instruments are notoriously treacherous, especially when administered to inpatients at high risk for suicide. A clinical suicide risk assessment with documented narrative should accompany the self-assessment. Any discrepancies between the two assessments require exploration with the patient. Some suicidal patients may reveal more on a form than in an interview (Sullivan and Bongar 2006). However, approximately 25% of patients at risk for suicide do not admit having suicidal ideation to the clinician (Robins 1981). The assumption that the patient is being truthful and wants to live cannot be blindly trusted. Some suicidal patients see the clinician and staff as the enemy and as an obstacle to their intent to die (Resnick 2002). Also the self-assessment may be falsified to obtain hospital discharge to pursue an unhindered suicide. Even if the patient answers truthfully, self-administered suicide scales are overly sensitive and lack specificity. For example, suicide risk factors are present in many depressed patients who do not attempt or complete suicide (Simon 2006).

Discrepancies can arise between checked-off suicide risk factors and the overall conclusion of suicide risk. For example, the clinician may check a number of moderate- and high-risk factors but conclude that the overall suicide risk is low or zero. The reasons for the discrepancy are not explained. The discrepancy is often the result of the clinician's denial and wishful thinking and the desire to reduce anxiety. Mechanical, obligatory form completion ill serves the patient and the clinician. Moreover, using a form puts the clinician on notice that a clinical assessment must also be performed. If forms are used, they should serve to encourage the clinician to perform a systematic suicide risk assessment instead of having the forms replacing the risk assessment.

General risk factors listed on the forms, derived from community-based psychological autopsy, cohort, and case-control studies, may not capture the suicidal patient's uniquely individual suicide risk and protective factors. For example, a schizophrenic patient with a severe stutter would begin to speak clearly whenever she would become acutely suicidal—at which point the patient would require immediate hospitalization. As she improved, the stutter would gradually return, allowing for a safe discharge. Stuttering is not a recognized suicide risk factor, except in this patient. Another example is that most forms do not take multicultural differences into account.

Assessment models can be used as teaching tools to help conceptualize the suicide risk assessment process (Simon 2006). However, heuristic models may encourage the use of forms instead of clinical assessment, unless a clear caveat is given.

Psychometric Scales and Measures: The Science

The Joint Commission (Joint Commission on Accreditation of Healthcare Organizations 2004) requires psychiatric facilities to use established tools to assess inpatients at risk for suicide. Each facility is responsible for developing its own suicide risk assessment protocol. This requirement has led to a proliferation of suicide risk assessment forms, some derived from a single-structured or semistructured clinical and research scales.

Commonly used standardized clinical scales include, for example, the Hamilton Rating Scale for Depression, the Beck Depression Inventory, and the Inventory of Depressive Symptomatology (Rush et al. 2008). Research scales with psychometric properties include the Columbia Suicide History Form, which elicits information about lifetime suicide attempts; Beck Scale for Suicide Ideation–characteristics of suicide ideation; Suicide Intent Scale–wish to die; Harkavy Asnis Suicide Survey–suicide ideation and behavior; and Beck Hopelessness Scale–negative attitudes about the future. Research scales and psychological instruments are not routinely used in clinical practice. However, the standardized suicide risk factor components of clinical and research scales are central to clinical assessment (e.g., suicide attempts, ideation, intent, hopelessness).

Psychological tests and suicide-risk scales may reveal suicidal ideation and elevated suicide risk in a patient whose initial clinical presentation may not trigger a suicide assessment (Sullivan and Bongar 2006). Tests and scales can contribute to an overall assessment that exposes biases and blind spots in clinical judgment. Generally, psychiatrists do not use psychological tests and suicide-risk scales in their suicide risk assessment. A survey by Zimmerman and McGlinchey (2008) in the United Kingdom revealed that only a minority of psychiatrists routinely used standardized measures to assess outcome when treating patients with depression and anxiety disorders. Psychiatrists did not routinely use scales because they did not find them clinically helpful and because they took too much time. Moreover, psychiatrists were not trained in the use of standardized measures.

The standard of care does not require that clinicians use psychological tests or checklists as part of the systematic assessment of suicide risk (Sullivan and Bongar 2006). A research or clinical scale cannot be a stand-alone substitute for clinical assessment of acute suicide risk (Rush et al. 2008). The scales and measures assess different domains of acute suicide risk. Even if all the scales were combined into a single risk assessment form, many other clinical risk factors would invariably be omitted. The variety of general and individual suicide risk factors cannot be captured by any form, no matter how elegantly constructed. Oquendo et al. (2003) discussed the utility and limitations of research instruments in assessing suicide risk.

Clinical Assessment

No single suicide risk assessment method has been empirically tested for reliability and validity (Simon 2006). Standard practice encompasses a wide range of reasoned clinical approaches (Simon 2006). The clinician's duty is to perform a competent suicide risk assessment using a reasonable method of assessment.

Use of assessment forms can increase the risk of suicide, when substituted for clinical assessment. Forms tend to be an event, whereas clinical assessment is a process. Some forms are completed at patient admission, others at discharge, or both. How often patients at risk for suicide must be clinically assessed depends on their risk status. The best scales cannot perform the integrative function of clinical assessment and judgment. Structured and semistructured suicide scales can, however, complement clinical assessment (American Psychiatric Association 2003).

Malone et al. (1995) found that semistructured screening instruments improved routine clinical assessment in the documentation and detection of lifetime suicidal behavior. A documented, brief narrative that describes the suicide risk and protective factors informing the overall assessment of risk is sufficient. Treatment and management interventions directed by the assessment and the effectiveness of the interventions should also be noted (Simon 2006).

Conclusion

Suicide risk assessment is a core competency. It is a process that identifies, prioritizes, and integrates suicide risk and protective factors into an overall assessment of the patient's suicide risk. Form completion is no substitute for spending the time necessary to know the patient. Assessment forms and checklists cannot perform this function. Using a suicide risk assessment form puts the clinician on notice that a competent assessment must be performed. Clinicians who use assessment forms must do more. Clinical assessment of suicide risk is still necessary. Clinical judgment cannot be abdicated in favor of filling out suicide risk assessment forms.

KEY CLINICAL CONCEPTS

- Forms are no substitute for spending time with the patient to get to know him or her.

- Forms and checklists, if used, must be accompanied by a documented narrative describing the suicide risk assessment process.

- Using a suicide risk assessment form places the clinician on notice that a competent assessment must be performed.

- Suicide risk assessment is a process of analysis and synthesis that identifies, prioritizes, and integrates acute and chronic risk and protective factors. Unaided assessment forms and checklists are *not* a substitute for this process.

- The greatest danger of forms and checklists is creating an illusion of clinical competence that preempts adequate suicide risk assessment.

References

American Psychiatric Association: Practice guidelines for the assessment and treatment of patients with suicidal behaviors. Am J Psychiatry 160 (suppl 11):1–60, 2003

Charles SC, Kennedy E: Defendant. New York, Free Press, 1985

Gabbard GO, Allison SE: Psychodynamic treatment, in The American Psychiatric Publishing Textbook of Suicide Assessment and Management. Edited by Simon RI, Hales RE. Washington, DC, American Psychiatric Publishing, 2006, pp 221–234

Gitlin M: Psychiatrists reactions to suicide, in The American Psychiatric Publishing Textbook of Suicide Assessment and Management. Edited by Simon RI, Hales RE. Washington, DC, American Psychiatric Publishing, 2006, pp 477–492

Joint Commission on Accreditation of Healthcare Organizations: Sentinel Event Statistics. December 31, 2004. Oak Brook Terrace, IL, Joint Commission on Accreditation of Healthcare Organizations, 2004

Malone KM, Katalin S, Corbill E, et al: Clinical assessment versus research methods in the assessment of suicidal behavior. Am J Psychiatry 152:1601–1607, 1995

Oquendo MA, Halbertham B, Mann JJ: Risk factors for suicidal behavior: the utility and limitations of research instruments, in Standardized Evaluation in Clinical Practice. Edited by First MB (Review of Psychiatry Series, Vol 22; Oldham JO and Riba MF, series eds). Washington DC, American Psychiatric Publishing, 2003, pp 103–130

Resnick PJ: Recognizing that the suicidal patient views you as an adversary. Curr Psychiatr 1:8, 2002

Robins E: The Final Months: Study of the Lives of 134 Persons Who Committed Suicide. New York, Oxford University Press, 1981

Rush AJ, First MB, Blacker E: Handbook of Psychiatric Measures: Suicide Risk Measures, 2nd Edition. Washington, DC, American Psychiatric Publishing, 2008

Scheiber SC, Kramer TS, Adamowski SE: Core Competencies for Psychiatric Practice: What Clinicians Need to Know (A Report of the American Board of Psychiatry and Neurology). Washington, DC, American Psychiatric Publishing, 2003, p 65

Simon RI: Suicide risk: assessing the unpredictable, in The American Psychiatric Publishing Textbook of Suicide Assessment and Management. Edited by Simon RI, Hales RE. Washington, DC, American Psychiatric Publishing, 2006, pp 1–32

Sullivan GR, Bongar B: Psychological testing in suicide risk management, in The American Psychiatric Publishing Textbook of Suicide Assessment and Management. Edited by Simon RI, Hales RE. Washington, DC, American Psychiatric Publishing, 2006, pp 177–196

Zimmerman M, McGlinchey JB: Why don't psychiatrists use scales to measure outcome when treating depressed patients? J Clin Psychiatry 69:1916–1919, 2008

CHAPTER 11

Imminent Suicide, Passive Suicidal Ideation, and Other Intractable Myths

EVIDENCE-BASED psychiatry is dispelling some of the entrenched myths, traditions, and uncritical acceptance of authority in clinical practice (Gray 2004). In the treatment of suicide patients, certain myths remain impervious to critical inquiry. In this chapter, three generally accepted myths that may undermine good clinical care of patients at risk for suicide are examined.

Imminent suicide is a euphemism for short-term prediction. It imposes an illusory time frame on an unpredictable act (Pokorny 1983). No short-term risk factor(s) identifies when, or even if, a patient will attempt or commit suicide (Harris et al. 2000; Simon 2004). Will the

Adapted with permission from Simon RI: "Imminent Suicide: The Illusion of Short-Term Prediction." *Suicide and Life-Threatening Behavior* 36:296–301, 2006.

patient attempt suicide in the next few minutes, hours, days, months, or years? In discussing the various time limits placed by clinicians on the accuracy of their predictions of dangerousness, Slovenko (1998, p. 303) states, "These time limits seemed to be pulled out of thin air." Actuarial analysis, a statistical measure, is useful in identifying diagnostic groups at higher risk for suicide compared with the general population (Addy 1992). But actuarial instruments do not address the imminence of suicide (Monahan et al. 2001).

"Imminence" defies definition. It is not a medical or psychiatric term. It is, however, in common clinical usage and firmly ensconced in clinical lore. Some clinicians assign arbitrary time limits for imminent suicide, although most time frames are vague (e.g., 24–48 hours, 1–3 weeks, 1 month). Hirschfield (1998) notes that "physicians must decide whether the risk is imminent (48 hours or less), short-term (within days or weeks), or long-term." He regards the risk of suicide "as imminent if the patient has expressed the intent to die, has a plan in mind, and has lethal means available." Rotheram (1987) suggests differentiating between imminent danger and suicide risk. The prediction of imminence is "modeled on methods used to evaluate or predict violence." Monahan (1981) defines imminent danger as occurring "within three days" of the prediction of a violent act. Fawcett et al. (1990) describe acute, short-term indicators that are statistically significant for suicide within 1 year of assessment. These authors attempt to define imminence, whereas other authors merely use the term incidentally (VandeCreek and Knapp 2000).

The term *imminent* is stated or implied in the substantive criteria of civil commitment statutes (Werth 2001). It is also found in duty-to-warn-and-protect case law and statutes or is imbedded in the language of the supporting statute or the court's opinion (*Mavroudis v. Superior Court for County of San Mateo* 1980).

Managed care protocols may require a recent suicide attempt to justify imminent risk criteria before approval of insurance benefits is granted for inpatient admission.

Standard of Care: Foreseeability Versus Prediction

Courts evaluate the psychiatrist's assessment and management of the patient who attempts or commits suicide to determine the reasonableness of the suicide risk assessment process and whether the patient's suicide attempt or completed suicide was foreseeable (Simon 2001). *Foreseeability* is a legal term of art, not a scientific construct. It is a commonsense, probabilistic concept.

There is an imperfect fit, however, between legal and psychiatric terminology. Foreseeability is legally defined as the reasonable anticipation that harm or injury is likely to result from certain acts or omissions (Black 1999). The law does not require defendants to "foresee events which are merely possible but only those that are reasonably foreseeable" (*Hairston v. Alexander Tank and Equip. Co.* 1984). Because suicide cannot be predicted, only the *risk* of suicide is foreseeable after adequate assessment (Simon 2002). Foreseeability should not be confused with the predictability of suicide. Imminence of suicide, another version of prediction, is not synonymous with foreseeability. The law does not assign a time limit for foreseeability. The lapse of time, by itself, does not bar recovery. It is only one factor to be weighed by the jury (*Naido v. Laird* 1988). Moreover, foreseeability is not the same as preventability. In hindsight, a suicide may have been preventable but not foreseeable at the time of evaluation (Meyer et al. 2010).

Involuntary Hospitalization

The substantive criteria for civil commitment of a patient require the presence of a mental illness and dangerousness to self or others (Simon and Shuman 2007). "Gravely disabled" may be subsumed under dangerousness to self. Dangerousness is a legal status, not a diagnosis or disposition. The concept of dangerousness has not been adequately explained by the courts. Courts tend to avoid precise meanings in defining dangerousness, preferring to keep the term vague in the common law tradition in order to preserve broad applicability to specific cases. Brooks (1978) divided dangerousness into five components: 1) nature of harm or conduct; 2) magnitude of harm; 3) probability; 4) imminence; and 5) frequency. Imminence is the only component that purports to address when a threatened violent act will occur. Nonetheless, imminence is also a legal term of art. It creates a legal fiction when it requires clinicians to adhere to legal requirements for which there are no professional standards of care.

The clinician is thus confronted with the stated or implied statutory requirement that the patient must be at imminent risk of suicide in order to meet the criteria for civil commitment (Melton et al. 1997). Melton et al. (1997) write, "Civil commitment is premised on *imminent* dangerousness; short-term, rather than long-term, danger to self or others is the focus." Some states require an "overt act" to bolster the likelihood that the danger is *imminent* rather than *distant* (American Psychiatric Association 2001, Section 4, Annotation 8).

Instead of feeling stymied or attempting to finesse the imminence criteria, the clinician may choose to err on the side of safeguarding the suicidal patient who needs involuntary hospitalization. The clinician only files a certification for involuntary hospitalization. The final decision to commit the patient is judicially determined. States have provisions in their commitment statutes granting psychiatrists and other mental health professionals immunity from liability when they use reasonable clinical judgment and act in good faith in petitioning for involuntary hospitalization (Simon 2004; see Chapter 7, "Patients at Acute and Chronic High Risk for Suicide: Crisis Management").

Professional organizations also use "imminent" language. For example, *The Principles of Medical Ethics With Annotations Especially Applicable to Psychiatry* (American Psychiatric Association 2001, Section 4, Annotation 8) advises psychiatrists about the limits of confidentiality with potentially violent patients: "Psychiatrists at times may find it necessary, in order to protect the patient or the community from *imminent* danger, to reveal confidential information disclosed by the patient" (Section 4, Annotation 8; emphasis added). Thus, in the Principles, psychiatrists are burdened with the impossible task of short-term prediction.

Managed Care Protocols

Some managed care organizations require that a patient be at "imminent" risk of suicide before approving coverage for inpatient admission. This situation frequently arises when psychiatrists or crisis counselors evaluate suicidal patients in the emergency department. Stating that the patient is imminently suicidal, by itself, does not open the insurance door to admission. Justification for this opinion is required—usually a recent overt suicide act or a suicide attempt within a specified period of time.

It is estimated that 8–25 suicide attempts occur for every completed suicide (National Institute of Mental Health 2003). Thus, on a statistical basis, a recent suicide attempt, however it is defined, does not indicate that a suicide attempt is "imminent." Many patients do not attempt suicide again. A high-risk suicidal patient who has made a near fatal suicide attempt in the distant past may be denied insurance coverage for not meeting the recent-overt-act requirement. The absence of a prior suicide attempt, recent or past, does not necessarily inform the clinician about the patient's current level of suicide risk.

Performing a systematic suicide risk assessment establishes the level of risk. A denial of coverage by a managed care organization that is based on the absence of a recent overt act (imminence) should not prevent admission of an acutely ill, high-risk suicidal patient. A doctor-to-doctor appeal should be pursued after the patient is admitted. It can be argued that imminence of suicide is not determinable and, hence, is not a valid criterion for admission. The clinician should emphasize that a recent overt act does not predict when or if a patient will attempt or commit suicide.

Hospital and clinic policies and procedures should avoid imposing a requirement that clinicians assess imminent self-harm—a requirement for which no standard of care exists. The term *imminent* or its equivalent (e.g., threatening, emergent) is also found in restraint and seclusion policies (American Psychiatric Association 1985). The justification for implementing seclusion and restraint procedures should be based on adequate risk assessment rather than the invocation of the talismanic word "imminent."

Assessing the Unpredictable

The improbability of predicting suicide in patients judged to be at imminent or short-term risk is based on a number of factors. Suicide is a rare event, even among suicidal patients identified to be at high risk. Patients who attempt or commit suicide are usually ambivalent about dying, some to the very last moment. Anecdotally, of 10 individuals who survived jumping from the Golden Gate Bridge, 8 changed their minds on the way down. Individuals in the act of attempting suicide have often been "talked down" from high places or persuaded to hand over loaded pistols. Suicide remains an uncertainty to the last moment.

A patient who makes the final decision to commit suicide may not do so immediately, but may wait for an opportune time (e.g., when a spouse or other family members are absent). A patient admitted to a psychiatric unit after a near-lethal suicide attempt may deny any intent to commit suicide while hospitalized. Between 15-minute checks or even under one-to-one supervision, the patient may seize a propitious moment to commit suicide (Fawcett et al. 2003).

Suicide risk may vary from minute to minute, hour to hour, or day to day. This makes any prediction about impending suicide illusory. Time attenuates the accuracy of suicide assessments, which are "here and now" judgments (Simon 2006). Therefore, suicide risk assessment must be a process, not an event.

Patients judged to be imminently suicidal are invariably acutely ill and at high risk for suicide. Merely noting that the patient is at imminent risk for suicide, without performing an adequate suicide risk assessment, deprives the clinician of the ability to identify, treat, and manage acute, patient-specific risk and protective factors. Clinicians who note that the patient is at imminent risk of suicide place themselves on notice that an adequate suicide risk assessment must be performed. Systematic suicide risk assessment identifies and prioritizes acute, modifiable, and treatable risk and protective factors that inform the overall treatment and safety management of the patient (Simon and Shuman 2009). The clinician can follow the patient's clinical course by assessing the response of these factors to treatment and safety management. Treating acute risk factors allows time for antidepressants to work in depressed patients. Anxiety, agitation, and insomnia often respond rapidly to treatment. Marshalling protective factors, such as involving supportive family members or partners, can help diminish suicide risk, which, in turn, allows the clinician to properly focus on patient treatment and safety management. "Imminence" is relegated to the realm of an illusion.

The judgment that a patient is at short-term risk for suicide should prompt the clinician to conduct systematic suicide risk assessments that inform continuing treatment and safety management. To borrow a phrase from Shakespeare, "imminence" is a word "full of sound and fury, signifying nothing" in the care of the patient at risk for suicide.

The Myth of Passive Suicidal Ideation

No evidence-based research supports the commonly held belief that "passive" suicidal ideation is less of a risk for suicide than "active" suicidal ideation. "Passive suicidal ideation" appears countless times in psychiatric records, articles, texts, guidelines, and clinical discourse. It is steeped in the lore and tradition of psychiatric practice.

Suicidal ideation, as discussed here, refers to thoughts about dying, either self-inflicted or by external factors. Although the method of suicide may be active or passive (e.g., firearm suicide versus suicide by cop), the goal is the same—terminating one's life. The assumption that passive suicidal ideation is a subset of suicidal ideation that is less severe, and thus reflects a low risk for suicide, is a falsely reassuring myth. Suicidal ideation, such as the wish to die during sleep, be killed by a vehicle, or develop terminal cancer, may seem innocuous, but it can be as deadly as thoughts of hanging. Presumably, a passive method of attempting suicide allows time for intervention, but methods can change without notice (Simon 2006). Suicidal ideation, without regard to "active" or "passive," is a moving target along a continuum of severity, reflecting constant change in the patient's underlying mental disorder and other risk factors (Isometsa and Lonnqvist 1998).

Suicidal ideation that expresses active or passive methods of suicide reflect psychodynamic, cultural, religious, and moral values as well as patient evasiveness, guardedness, denial, and other factors. Passive suicidal ideation may contain potential protective factors, such as supportive family or coping skills, that are best evaluated separately within the overall suicide risk assessment. Otherwise, the clinician may prematurely conclude that no further risk assessment is necessary.

"Fleeting" suicidal ideation, a frequent companion of "passive" suicidal ideation, also requires careful evaluation. Hall et al. (1999), in a study of 100 patients who made severe suicide attempts, found that 29 of the patients had serious, persistent suicidal ideation before they attempted suicide. However, 69 patients reported only fleeting or no suicidal ideation before their attempt.

Reynolds et al. (1996) assessed the clinical correlates of active suicidal ideation versus passive death wishes in elderly patients with recurrent major depression. Their data challenged the utility of distinguishing active and passive suicidal ideation. They also noted that the patient's ideation can change from passive to active during an episode of illness. They recommended that clinicians be no less vigilant with patients expressing passive suicidal ideation.

The Scale for Suicide Ideation, and the later version, Beck Scale for Suicide Ideation (Rush et al. 2008), rate "passive suicidal attempt" as

0   "would take precautions to save life"
1   "would leave life/death to chance (e.g., carelessly crossing a busy street)"
2   "would avoid steps necessary to save or maintain life (e.g., diabetic ceasing to take insulin)"

Although the Beck scales have psychometric properties (reliability and validity), no scale, or portion thereof, can substitute for thorough clinical assessment of suicidal ideation. If used, ratings scales or checklists of suicidal ideation should alert the clinician that he or she must thoroughly assess the nature and severity of this crucial symptom of suicide risk.

Case Example

A 56-year-old business executive is brought to an emergency room by his wife. The patient's business is facing bankruptcy. He is unable to go to the office and face his employees. The patient cannot sleep or eat and spends most of the day laying on the couch and crying. The patient's wife threatens her husband with separation if he does not seek psychiatric treatment.

The patient tells the emergency room psychiatrist, "I am stressed but have no intention of hurting myself. I love my wife and kids too much to put them through that." The patient does admit to having wishes to die in his sleep but says, "I can't sleep anyway." The patient's wife found a loaded gun in the glove compartment of his car. The patient states that the "gun is for my protection." He angrily denies any suicidal ideation and protests, "I do not need to be here." The patient's wife insists that he be treated, stating "I will not take my husband home in his condition."

The patient refuses psychiatric hospitalization but changes his mind when confronted with involuntary hospitalization. He admits that, unknown to his wife, he recently purchased a $2 million life insurance policy and made funeral arrangements. He planned to kill himself with his revolver. A thorough suicide risk assessment reveals a number of risk factors that place the patient at acute, high risk for suicide.

"Passive suicidal ideation" does not inform suicide risk assessment; it merely casts a spell of complacency upon the clinician. It is not a valid clinical distinction. Clinicians do not think of active or passive anxiety, depression, or insomnia. Similarly, suicidal ideation should not be split into active and passive. To do so undermines the singular importance of suicidal ideation as a unitary risk factor for suicide. For too long, the myth has existed in clinical practice that passive suicidal ideation is benign, thus creating a false sense that the patient is at little or no risk for suicide. Thus, suicide risk assessment may be prematurely suspended.

Suicidal ideation must be carefully assessed, not labeled. Passive suicidal ideation should not deter the clinician from performing competent suicide risk assessments. Suicidal ideation that contains passive or active methods of attempting suicide expresses one goal—the termination of life.

When the Suicidal Patient Calls: The Myth of True Emergency[1]

Psychiatrists and other mental health professionals leave voice mail messages on their office phones advising patients what to do in case of an emergency. When a suicidal patient in crisis calls the psychiatrist and hears the recorded message: "If you have a 'true' emergency, go to your nearest emergency room or call 911," the patient's risk of suicide may increase.

Psychiatrists and other mental health professionals must be accessible to their suicidal patients or must provide for adequate coverage in their absence. The psychiatrist may be the only person with whom the suicidal patient has a life-affirming relationship.

What exactly is a "true" emergency? Who can define it? "True" emergency is devoid of meaning—a myth. But the suicidal patient may perceive the true message as "Don't bother me!" The "true" emergency message erects a barrier between the patient and the psychiatrist. Does this message, which is now increasingly heard, reflect an erosion of the doctor-patient relationship wrought by changes in mental health care delivery? Is it also a misguided effort at risk management?

Emergency Accessibility

Leaving the message, "If you have a 'true' emergency, go to your nearest emergency room" or the variant "call 911," leaves the patient with

---

[1] Adapted with permission from "True Emergency? Suicidal Patients' Access to their Psychiatrists." *Psychiatric Times,* March 2008.

few options. Suicidal patients are often reluctant to call 911. The police and rescue squad will arrive at their door with sirens blaring. A crowd of inquisitive neighbors will gather. The street scene is embarrassing and humiliating. The patient may be too impaired or unwilling to follow the instructions, instead choosing to attempt or complete suicide.

The general hospital emergency department is the main venue for suicidal patients requiring immediate care. In a consultative model of care, the patient is first evaluated by the emergency department physician. If psychiatric consultation is requested, the crisis counselor usually sees the patient first. An attending psychiatrist is available on call for consultation, usually by phone. In most instances, a general hospital's emergency department provides adequate care. The emergency department experience, however, can add to the patient's distress. Psychiatric patients report enduring long periods of time waiting to be evaluated in busy general hospital emergency departments. For example, the patient may not be seen for hours or even for a day or more. Hours of waiting in mental misery confirms the patient's feelings of hopeless abandonment, increasing suicide risk. A suicidal patient with agitated depression or a psychotic patient with auditory hallucinations commanding suicide may leave the emergency department before being seen and then attempt or complete suicide.

Psychiatric Emergency Services (PES), staffed by psychiatrists and a full complement of other mental health professionals, are usually based at large university medical centers or schools. They are open 24 hours a day, 7 days a week, and provide "full service," comprehensive emergency psychiatric services (Breslow 2002).

Generally, the phone call to the patient is an intermediary step in determining an initial course of action. The psychiatrist may be able to assess the severity of a known patient's suicidal crisis by phone and, if necessary, to arrange an emergency appointment. If possible, the patient may be managed by means other than referral to the emergency department. A return-call from the psychiatrist can stabilize a suicidal patient long enough for the patient to be seen the same or next day. Thus, therapeutic alliance is preserved and strengthened.

It may be necessary to send a suicidal patient in need of immediate care to the emergency department, or the patient may go to the emergency department without calling the psychiatrist. In the former instance, the psychiatrist can determine whether the patient is able to go to the emergency department alone or needs to be accompanied. The suicidal patient may be so disturbed that he or she is unable to come to the psychiatrist's office or speak coherently to the psychiatrist on the phone. The psychiatrist should try to enlist the assistance of others (e.g., family member, partner, friend, or police) before sending the patient to the emergency department. The psychiatrist may have no recourse but to call 911 or community crisis management services. A phone call to the psychiatric emergency services or general hospital emergency department in advance of the patient's arrival will alert and inform the staff about the suicidal patient. It also may help decrease the waiting time in the emergency department.

The psychiatrist or covering clinician who is informed about suicidal patients that might call must be available to respond within a reasonable period of time. What is reasonable? Although hard-and-fast rules do not exist, if possible, an emergency call from a suicidal patient should be responded to within the hour. For a patient in a suicide crisis, even waiting an hour may seem like an eternity.

In solo practice, the psychiatrist or covering clinician has to be accessible to calls from suicidal patients 24 hours a day, 7 days a week, by cell phone, pager, or other means of direct communication. Twenty-four-hour coverage for patient emergencies is an established medical practice and standard of care. Psychiatrists in group practice or institutional settings have on-call schedules that provide continuous coverage for patients. Some psychiatrists provide their home phone number to a patient during a period of increased risk of suicide.

The "Opinions of the Ethics Committee on The Principles of Medical Ethics With Annotations Especially Applicable to Psychiatry" (American Psychiatric Association 2001, Section 1-AA) takes a firm position on emergency coverage of patients:

> **Question A:** One of our members is concerned that psychiatrists in his area do not routinely check in with their answering machines after hours, leave no number where they may be reached, or leave a message for patients to contact the local emergency room in case of emergency. Is this member's concern about the ethics of these psychiatrists warranted?

> **Answer:** Yes. Ethical psychiatrists are obliged to render competent care to their patients. That competent care would include either being available for emergencies at all times or making appropriate arrangements. Certainly, a message telling patients to call an emergency room is not adequate coverage. Even in rather stable practices, in-

cluding analytic practices with relatively stable patients, emergencies do arise. Care must be taken that, if and when such emergencies do arise, the patient is not abandoned. (September 1993)

Patient Education: A Pre-arranged Safety Plan

With the current limitations on access to hospital services, most patients at risk for suicide, even some who are chronically at high risk, are treated as outpatients. Some psychiatrists provide and discuss with new patients a safety protocol to be followed in an emergency. The spirit of the discussion is "We're in it together." Alliance building encourages the patient, who might not do so otherwise, to call the psychiatrist during a crisis. Psychiatrists explain how they can be reached in an emergency. The psychiatrist or covering clinician may not be able to return the patient's call within the time that an acutely suicidal patient needs immediate assistance. In the pre-arranged plan, the patient will leave a message with a phone number for the psychiatrist that he or she has gone to a safe holding place to await the psychiatrist's call (e.g., home, family, friend, or other) or if necessary to a predetermined emergency department. If a psychiatric emergency services facility is accessible to the patient, the address and phone number should be provided. The psychiatrist will call the emergency department at the first opportunity to assist in the patient's assessment and management.

Some patients at risk for suicide do not have family, partners, friends, or other supportive resources. If unable to wait for a callback from the psychiatrist, the patient should be provided with suicide prevention hot lines as a source of assistance. The National Suicide Prevention Lifeline (1-800-273-TALK) can refer the patient to local hotlines and other sources of help. The website is www.suicidepreventionlifeline.org.

Patients at risk for suicide need to have hotline phone numbers readily available. The patient may not be able to find a hotline phone number during a suicide crisis. Hotline phone numbers must be verified as correct before being given to the patient. The psychiatrist should document the pre-arranged safety plan, including the patient's understanding and agreement.

The standard of care requires that psychiatrists or their designees be accessible to suicidal patients and must respond within a reasonable time. This also applies to psychiatrists and psychotherapists providing conjoint or "split treatment." Each is individually, as well as jointly, clinically responsible for the patient (Meyer and Simon 2006).

Case Example[2]

While a psychiatrist is having dinner with her family at a restaurant, she receives an emergency page from a patient who is at chronic high risk for suicide. The psychiatrist discussed with the patient at the beginning of treatment how she could be reached if the patient became suicidal. The psychiatrist calls the patient, who screams, "My bastard boyfriend dumped me. I want to die!" The patient has bought a gun and intends to use it. The patient abruptly hangs up. The psychiatrist calls the patient repeatedly but the line is constantly busy.

The psychiatrist calls 911. The rescue squad and police arrive at the patient's apartment. The door is barricaded. The police break it down. The patient refuses to tell the police where the gun is hidden. A search reveals that the gun is in a kitchen cabinet. The patient vehemently denies that she is suicidal, stating, "It was just a fleeting thought." The patient leaves the apartment with a coat over her head to avoid "nosy neighbors." The police take the patient to a general hospital emergency department.

The patient is initially uncooperative in the emergency department, only reluctantly providing her psychiatrist's name and phone number. The emergency department crisis counselor calls the psychiatrist to obtain information about the patient. The psychiatrist states that the patient has been treated for over a year for bipolar disorder II and borderline personality disorder. The patient, now age 36 years, made a serious suicide attempt by medication overdose at age 25 years, following the break-up of a romantic relationship. The patient has been at moderate to high chronic risk for suicide over the years, requiring hospitalization during acute suicidal episodes, usually precipitated by a failed, abusive relationship. The psychiatrist informs the crisis counselor that the patient is receiving once-a-week psychotherapy and provides the names of medications she is taking.

The crisis counselor and psychiatrist agree that the patient needs to be admitted to the psychiatric inpatient unit. The patient initially refuses hospital admission. But after the psychiatrist speaks to her by phone, the patient agrees to be voluntarily admitted. The patient's psychiatrist calls the admitting psychiatrist to provide additional clinical information. She later finishes her take-home dinner.

---

[2]Case disguised to protect patient identity and ensure confidentiality.

Abandonment

Abandonment is legally defined as negligently failing to attend a patient, absent the proper termination of the doctor-patient relationship (Simon and Shuman 2007). It may either be overt or implied (e.g., failure to attend, monitor, or observe the patient). Some courts have expanded the concept of abandonment to include situations in which delay and inattention in providing care caused the patient injury, termed *constructive abandonment* (i.e., as though actual abandonment had occurred) (Mains 1985). For example, in *Bolles v. Kinton* (1928), the court stated that a physician cannot, without sufficient notice, discharge a patient by simply not attending the patient. Other courts have found abandonment when psychiatrists were inaccessible to patients, particularly if a crisis was occurring or if the crisis was foreseeable. The following have been construed by courts as negligent acts amounting to abandonment:

- Failure to provide patients with a way to contact the psychiatrist between sessions
- Failure to provide adequate clinical coverage when the psychiatrist is away from practice

When a psychiatrist agrees to treat a patient, a psychiatrist-patient relationship is formed, creating the duty to provide treatment to the patient as is necessary (Fochtmann 2006). The accessibility of the psychiatrist to the suicidal patient who calls for help can prevent a suicide attempt or completion. Psychiatrists' availability to their patients can also result in fewer emergency calls. Patients are less anxious when they know they can reach their psychiatrist. The patient who calls frequently claiming a suicidal crisis when none exists is rare.

When a psychiatrist or the covering clinician is inaccessible to a suicidal patient who calls and subsequently attempts or completes suicide, the psychiatrist may be sued for abandonment. A distraught, acutely suicidal patient may not be able or willing to follow the instructions of a recorded message that states, "If you have a 'true' emergency, please go to the nearest emergency room or call 911." The patient may conclude, "Nobody cares, not even my psychiatrist."

Risk Management

As a risk management strategy, leaving a "true" emergency message is worse than useless; it is irrelevant and gratuitous. It is likely to invite a lawsuit more than to prevent one. Suicidal patients know that they can always go to an emergency department. In a crisis, they want to speak to their therapists.

Effective risk management depends on adequate documentation of an emergency call from a suicidal patient. The following information should be documented: date and time of the patient's call, nature of the emergency, discussion with the patient, immediate interventions implemented, and follow-up actions taken (Simon 2004). Clinical care that conforms to the standard of care regarding emergency accessibility can help provide a solid defense against a claim of abandonment.

In their absence, psychiatrists should arrange for adequate coverage of their practices by similarly qualified clinicians (Simon and Hales 2006). The covering clinician needs to be informed about suicidal patients who might call. In addition, the covering clinician should respond to patient calls in a timely manner and, if necessary, see the patient for an emergency appointment. The covering clinician also has malpractice exposure for abandonment, if failure to attend the patient causes the patient harm.

Conclusion

Imminent suicide is the illusion that suicide can be predicted, especially in the near term. No suicide risk factors can predict when or if a patient will attempt or commit suicide.

The second myth is that suicidal ideation is binary. Splitting suicidal ideation into active and passive creates the illusion that passive suicidal ideation is innocuous.

Finally, leaving a "true emergency" message for patients in crises, especially suicidal patients, is flawed risk management. It is likely to invite a lawsuit more than prevent one. Patients in suicidal crisis who are unable to contact their treater may feel abandoned, thus increasing their risk for suicide.

KEY CLINICAL CONCEPTS

- The term *imminent* is a euphemism for short-term prediction. No short-term suicide risk factors exist that can predict when or if a patient will attempt suicide.

- "Imminent suicide" should never be used in place of an adequate suicide risk assessment.

- No evidence-based research supports the belief that "passive" suicidal ideation is less of a risk for suicide that "active" suicidal ideation. In both cases, the intent is to die, but in passive suicidal ideation, it is by indirect means.

- The clinician should not require patients at risk for suicide to discern the meaning of "true emergency," when they call for assistance.

- When clinicians undertake the care of a suicidal patient, they must be accessible in emergencies or provide appropriate coverage.

References

Addy C: Statistical concepts of prediction, in Assessment and Prediction of Suicide. Edited by Maris RW, Berman AL, Maltsberger JT, et al. New York, Guilford, 1992, pp 218–222

American Psychiatric Association: The Psychiatric Uses of Seclusion and Restraint (Task Force Report No 22). Washington, DC, American Psychiatric Association, 1985

American Psychiatric Association: Principles of Medical Ethics With Annotations Especially Applicable to Psychiatry. Washington, DC, American Psychiatric Association, 2001

Black HC: Black's Law Dictionary, 7th Edition. St. Paul, MN, West Publishing Group, 1999

Bolles v Kinton, 83 Colo.147, 153, 263, p 28 (1928)

Breslow RE: Structure and function of psychiatric emergency services, in Emergency Psychiatry. Edited by Allen MH (Review of Psychiatry Series, Vol 21; Oldham JM and Riba MB, series eds). Washington, DC, American Psychiatric Publishing, 2002, pp 1–31

Brooks AD: Notes on defining the "dangerousness" of the mentally ill, in Dangerous Behavior: A Problem in Law and Mental Health (DHEW Publ No ADM-78-563). Edited by Frederick CJ. Rockville, MD, National Institute of Mental Health, 1978, pp 37–60

Fawcett J, Scepter WA, Fogg L, et al: Time-related predictors of suicide in major affective disorder. Am J Psychiatry 147:1189–1194, 1990

Fawcett J, Busch KA, Jacobs DG: Clinical correlates of inpatient suicide. J Clin Psychiatry 64:14–19, 2003

Fochtmann LJ: Emergency services, in The American Psychiatric Publishing Textbook of Suicide Assessment and Management. Edited by Simon RI, Hales RE. Washington, DC, American Psychiatric Publishing, 2006, pp 381–400

Gray GE: Concise Guide to Evidence-Based Psychiatry. Washington, DC, American Psychiatric Publishing, 2004

Hairston v Alexander Tank and Equip Co, 310 NC 227, 234, 311, SE2d 559, 565, 1984

Hall RC, Platt DE, Hall RC: Suicide risk assessment: a review of risk factors for suicide in 100 patients who made severe suicide attempts. Evaluation of suicide risk in a time of managed care. Psychosomatics 40:18–27, 1999

Harris MR, Holman J, Bates AA, et al: Completed suicides and emergency psychiatric evaluations: the Louisville experience. J Ky Med Assoc 98:210–212, 2000

Hirschfield RM: The suicidal patient. Hosp Pract 33:127–128, 1998

Isometsa ET, Lonnqvist JK: Suicide attempts preceding completed suicide. Br J Psychiatry 173:531–535, 1998

Mains J: Medical abandonment. Med Trial Tech Q 31:306–328, 1985

Mavroudis v Superior Court for County of San Mateo, 102 Cal3d 594 at 400, 162 Cal Rptr 724 at 730, 1980

Melton GB, Petrila J, Poythress NG, et al: Psychological Evaluations for the Courts, 2nd Edition. New York, Guilford, 1997

Meyer DJ, Simon RI: Split treatment, in The American Psychiatric Publishing Textbook of Suicide Assessment and Management. Edited by Simon RI, Hales RE. Washington, DC, American Psychiatric Publishing, 2006, pp 235–251

Meyer DJ, Simon RI, Shuman DW: Psychiatric malpractice and the standard of care, in The American Psychiatric Publishing Textbook of Forensic Psychiatry, 2nd Edition. Edited by Simon RI, Gold LH. Washington, DC, American Psychiatric Publishing, 2010, pp 207–226

Monahan J: Predicting Violent Behavior. Beverly Hills, CA, Sage, 1981

Monahan J, Steadman H, Silver E, et al: Rethinking Risk Assessment: The MacArthur Study of Mental Disorder and Violence. New York, Oxford University Press, 2001

Naido v Laird, 539 A 2d 1064 (Del. Super. Ct.), 1988

National Institute of Mental Health: Suicide. Available at: http://www.nimh. nih.gov/research/suifact.htm. Accessed January 3, 2003.

Pokorny AD: Prediction of suicide in psychiatric patients: report of a prospective study. Arch Gen Psychiatry 40:249–257, 1983

Reynolds CF, Frank E, Sack J, et al: Suicide in elderly depressed patients: is active vs. passive suicidal ideation a clinically valid distinction? Am J Geriatr Psychiatry 4:197–207, 1996

Rotheram MF: Evaluation of imminent danger for suicide among youth. Am J Orthopsychiatry 17:102–110, 1987

Rush AJ, First MB, Blacker E: Handbook of Psychiatric Measures: Suicide Risk Measures, 2nd Edition. Washington, DC, American Psychiatric Publishing, 2008, pp 242–244

Simon RI: Psychiatry and Law for Clinicians, 3rd Edition. Washington, DC, American Psychiatric Publishing, 2001

Simon RI: Suicide risk assessment: what is the standard of care? J Am Acad Psychiatry Law 30:340–344, 2002

Simon RI: Assessing and Managing Suicide Risk: Guidelines for Clinically Based Risk Management. Washington, DC, American Psychiatric Publishing, 2004

Simon RI: Suicide risk assessment: assessing the unpredictable, in The American Psychiatric Publishing Textbook of Suicide Assessment and Management. Edited by Simon RI, Hales RE. Washington, DC, American Psychiatric Publishing, 2006, pp 1–32

Simon RI, Hales RE (eds): The American Psychiatric Publishing Textbook of Suicide Assessment and Management. Washington, DC, American Psychiatric Publishing, 2006

Simon RI, Shuman DW: Clinical Manual of Psychiatry and Law. Washington, DC, American Psychiatric Publishing, 2007

Simon RI, Shuman DW: Clinical-legal issues of psychiatry, in Comprehensive Textbook of Psychiatry, 8th Edition. Edited by Sadock BJ, Sadock VA. Philadelphia, PA, Lippincott Williams & Williams, 2009, pp 4427–4438

Slovenko R: Psychotherapy and Confidentiality. Springfield, IL, Charles C Thomas, 1998

VandeCreek L, Knapp S: Risk management and life threatening behavior. J Clin Psychology 56:1335–1351, 2000

Werth JL: U.S. involuntary mental health commitment statutes: requirements for perceived to be a potential harm to self. Suicide Life Threat Behav 31:348–357, 2001

CHAPTER 12

Quality Assurance Review of Suicide Risk Assessments

Reality and Remedy

SUICIDE risk assessment is a core competency that the psychiatrist must possess (Scheiber et al. 2003). A competent suicide assessment identifies modifiable and treatable risk and protective factors that inform patient treatment and safety management (Simon 2002). A clinical axiom holds that there are two kinds of psychiatrists—those who have had patients commit suicide and those who will. Patient suicide is an occupational hazard. Psychiatrists, unlike other medical specialists, do not often experience patient deaths, except by suicide.

Psychiatrists frequently assess suicidal patients who present life-threatening emergencies. Unlike other physicians, psychiatrists do not have laboratory tests and sophisticated diagnostic instruments to assess patients at risk for suicide. For example, when evaluating an emergency cardiac patient, the clinician can order a number of diagnostic tests and procedures such as electrocardiogram, serial enzymes, imaging, and catheterization. The psychiatrist's diagnostic instrument is competent suicide risk assessment.

No single suicide risk assessment method has been empirically tested for reliability and validity (Simon 2006). Standard practice encompasses a range of reasoned clinical approaches to suicide risk assessment. From a risk management perspective, the law does not require ideal, best practices, or even good care. The clinician's duty is to provide reasonable risk assessment (Simon 2002).

The Reality

A review of suicide cases in litigation reveals an absence of documented suicide risk assessments (Simon 2002). Instead, a note containing "NO SI, HI, CFS" (no suicide ideation, homicidal ideation, contracts for safety) often masquerades as a suicide risk assessment. A layperson could just as well conduct such an assessment.

The situation is no different with regard to quality assurance reviews. Repeated requests for documented suicide risk assessments have proved fruitless. Substandard suicide risk assessment is the second-most common root cause of inpatient suicides, contributing to approximately 85% of inpatient suicides (Sokolov et al. 2006). Documented suicide risk assessments are a core measure of quality care.

Why, then, are documented suicide risk assessments a rarity? When this question is posed to colleagues, the following is a sample of the reasons given:

1. The clinician has not learned how to perform an adequate suicide risk assessment.
2. Risk and protective factors may be identified during the course of an evaluation but not prioritized and integrated into a standalone clinical judgment of overall suicide risk that informs patient treatment and management.
3. The clinician does not do suicide risk assessments commonly in inpatient settings, delegating the task to others.
4. The clinician performs adequate suicide risk assessments but fails to document assessments.

5. The clinician experiences anxiety in the treatment of the suicidal patient, which creates denial and minimization of risk, resulting in inadequate assessment.
6. The clinician worries that if the assessment is wrong and the patient attempts or completes suicide, documenting the risk assessment process creates liability exposure.
7. The clinician who treats patients in an inpatient setting with rapid patient turnover and short length of stay or in a busy outpatient medication management practice may not take or have the time necessary to perform a competent suicide risk assessment.
8. Assessment forms may be robotically checked off, without a narrative describing the suicide assessment process.
9. So-called "suicide prevention contracts" supplant competent suicide risk assessments.
10. The clinician relies on intuitive, "gut" assessment of suicide risk.

Time, money, inadequate training, and litigation fears can combine to negatively influence adequate suicide risk assessment and documentation. The fear of becoming embroiled in a malpractice suit, if a patient attempts or completes suicide, can engender inappropriate defensive practices (Simon and Shuman 2009; see Chapter 13, "Therapeutic Risk Management of the Patient at Risk for Suicide"). Countertransference hate of a suicidal patient who provokes anxiety in the psychiatrist can result in inadequate risk assessment and treatment (Gabbard and Allison 2006). Most psychiatrists have not been formally trained on how to conduct suicide risk assessments. The clinician must do much more than just rely on a *sense* of suicide risk in the air or on a "gut" feeling. It is generally assumed that clinicians will somehow acquire this knowledge in the course of their clinical practices.

As the internist must be trained to assess the emergency cardiac patient, so the psychiatrist must be trained to competently assess the suicidal patient. The core competence necessary to perform suicide risk assessments is difficult to obtain through unaided clinical experience alone. Learning how to perform competent suicide risk assessments must begin during psychiatric residency. Lectures, tutorials, and, especially, case conferences that follow patients at suicide risk during the course of treatment are essential.

An extensive psychiatric literature exists on suicide, but relatively little has been written on the topic of suicide risk assessment. This is beginning to change. McNeil et al. (2008) demonstrated that structured clinical training in evidence-based risk assessment can improve the documentation of assessment and management of suicidal patients. The American Psychiatric Association's "Practice Guideline for the Assessment and Treatment of Patients With Suicidal Behaviors" (American Psychiatric Association 2003) is an excellent informational source regarding the conduct of suicide risk assessment.

The Remedy

Forms and checklists are not effective substitutes for clinical assessment (Simon 2009). Generally, self-assessment instruments cannot be relied on, because guarded or deceptive suicidal patients will not answer honestly. Some patients, however, may reveal more about suicide risk on self-assessment forms than at the clinical interview (Sullivan and Bongar 2006). No psychological tests exist that can predict suicide (Sullivan and Bongar 2006). Assessment forms and checklists often omit evidence-based general risk factors. Some checklists contain items that are not even recognized risk factors for suicide. Also, unique, individual, suicide risk factors are not present on assessment forms. The "know your patient imperative" is absent. Checking off forms robotically is not a credible risk assessment. If litigation ensues following a patient's suicide, the plaintiff's attorney will invariably point out to the jury the suicide risk factors that the deceased patient manifested but were not on the form (see Chapter 10, "Suicide Risk Assessment Forms: Clinician Beware").

As noted earlier, there are numerous suicide risk assessment methods (Simon 2002). Suicide risk assessment is a process of analysis and synthesis, which requires identifying, prioritizing, and integrating multiple risk and protective factors into an overall clinical judgment of risk. Figure 12–1 is a conceptual model for conducting suicide risk assessment. Clinicians, however, may construct their own approach to suicide risk assessment on the basis of their training, clinical experience, and their familiarity with the suicide literature. The singular importance of suicide risk assessments necessitates that the assessment process be documented as a separate narrative paragraph in the psychiatric evaluation or in the progress notes. Armed with the ability to perform competent suicide risk assessments, the psychiatrist can con-

	Risk factors	Protective factors	
	EXAMPLES:	**EXAMPLES:**	
Acute	• Depression • Anxiety • Insomnia	• Therapeutic alliance • Child under age 18 at home • Spousal/family support	Current
Chronic	• Suicide attempt(s) • Family history of suicide • Childhood abuse	• Coping/survival skills • Moral/religious beliefs • Capacity for relationships	Lifelong

Instructions:

1. Complete all grid boxes to form an overall clinical judgment of suicide risk.

2. Treat acute risk factors and mobilize protective factors.

FIGURE 12–1.   Conceptual model for suicide risk assessment.

fidently manage the patient at risk for suicide, one of the more complex, difficult, and challenging clinical tasks in psychiatry.

In a "Sentinel Event Alert" the Joint Commission (1998) conducted a root cause analysis of 65 inpatient suicides. Failure to perform adequate suicide risk assessments was found to be a root cause in the suicides. Revising suicide risk assessment procedures was noted as an important risk reduction strategy. Effective January 1, 2007, The Joint Commission required psychiatric facilities to use established tools to assess patients at risk for suicide (The Joint Commission 2009).

What is the remedy? First, regular chart review for ensuring documented, competent, suicide risk assessments can be performed by quality assurance committees on inpatient services or similarly constituted committees in outpatient settings. Consensus criteria for evaluating the adequacy of documented suicide risk assessments must be determined first. The assessment framework will vary according to the clinical setting and the clinical staff's experiences with suicidal patients. Once established, the criteria can be modified over time, as necessary. Second, The Joint Commission (2010) requires that objective measures of the quality of a physician's performance be established for recredentialing. Suicide risk assessment is an important measure of

Suicide risk assessment guideline

- Assessed suicide risk and protective factors*
- Documented suicide risk assessment
- Treated acute suicide risk factors
- Mobilized protective factors
- Implemented safety management interventions based on the patient's suicide risk assessment
- Documented decision-making rationale
- Assessed effectiveness of interventions

*Admission, discharge, and significant changes in the patient's clinical status.

FIGURE 12–2.   **Suicide risk assessment quality assurance review**

clinical competence for periodic chart review. Third, a "Suicide Risk Assessment Guideline" (see Figure 12–2) can be included in the medical chart. The guideline is not a suicide risk assessment instrument. Instead, it encourages the clinician to perform a systematic suicide risk assessment. Periodic chart review will determine if the suicide risk assessment guideline is improving the clinician's quality of assessment. Figure 12–3 is a companion to the guideline describing the suicide risk assessment process. Unless there is a continuing review and oversight process for compliance with standard suicide risk assessment measures, risk assessment of suicidal patients will likely continue to be sporadic, idiosyncratic, and inadequate.

Conclusion

Finally, there is no foolproof way of ensuring that competent suicide risk assessments will be performed. The unfortunate reality is that documented suicide risk assessments are rare, if in fact they are actually conducted or conducted competently. As with other measures of physician quality performance, conducting competent suicide risk assessments must be subject to continuing, consistent, monitoring.

The suicide risk assessment process

A. Purpose: Identify treatable and modifiable suicide risk and protective factors that guide the patient's treatment and management.
B. Assessment: There is no standard suicide risk assessment methodology. One way of conceptualizing assessment is to divide acute and chronic risk factors into 5 categories: 1) individual, 2) clinical, 3) interpersonal, 4) situation, and 5) demographic. Another conceptual method is demonstrated in Figure 12–1. Acute risk factors include the patient's symptoms and stressful circumstances that require immediate clinical attention. Assess both suicide risk and protective factors. Suicide risk assessment is a process of analysis and synthesis that requires identifying, prioritizing, and integrating risk and protective factors into an overall clinical judgment of suicide risk. It is a "here and now" assessment that needs frequent updating.
C. Documentation: Record all suicide risk assessments. The standard of care requires that clinicians document important assessments and interventions. Documentation is essential to patient care. It supports good patient care and explains clinical decision-making. Documentation is also good risk management. Because of the importance of suicide risk assessment, it should be so identified and recorded as a separate narrative paragraph in the clinical evaluation or progress note.
D. Treatment: Identify and prioritize acute risk and protective factors for aggressive treatment and safety management. Suicide risk assessments are performed on admission, on discharge, and at significant changes in the patient's clinical status.
E. Safety management: Suicide risk assessment guides clinical judgment regarding the patient's safety requirements. Perform and document risk assessments that support changes in the patient's level of safety management.
F. Decision-making rationale: Document a brief narrative summary describing how the suicide risk assessment informed treatment and safety management decisions. Avoid conclusory statements such as "low, moderate, or high risk," unless it is supported by the suicide risk assessment.
G. Effectiveness of interventions: Assess and document the patient's response to treatment and management of suicide risk and protective factors.

FIGURE 12–3.   The suicide risk assessment process.

KEY CLINICAL CONCEPTS

- Suicide risk assessment is a core competency that the psychiatrist must possess.

- The singular importance of suicide risk assessments requires that the assessment process be documented as a separate narrative paragraph in the psychiatric evaluation or in the medical record.

- Regular chart review for ensuring documented, competent, suicide risk assessments can be performed by quality assurance committees on inpatient services or similarly constituted committees in outpatient settings.

- Documented suicide risk assessments are rare, if in fact they are actually conducted or conducted competently.

- The suicide risk assessment quality assurance review and the conceptual model for suicide risk assessment are clinical tools to assist and improve the conduct of suicide risk assessments.

References

American Psychiatric Association: Practice guideline for the assessment and treatment of patients with suicidal behaviors. Am J Psychiatry 160 (suppl 11):1–60, 2003

Gabbard GO, Allison SE: Psychodynamic treatment, in The American Psychiatric Publishing Textbook of Suicide Assessment and Management. Edited by Simon RI, Hales RE. Washington, DC, American Psychiatric Publishing, 2006, pp 221–234

The Joint Commission: Sentinel Event Alert: Inpatient suicides: recommendations for prevention. November 6, 1998. Available at: http://www.jointcommission. org/SentinelEvents/Sentineleventalert/sea_7.htm. Accessed February 1, 2010.

The Joint Commission: 2009 National Patient Safety Goals. January 1, 2009. Available at: http://www.jcrinc.com/common/PDFs/fpdfs/pubs/pdfs/JCReqs/JCP-07-08-S1.pdf. Accessed February 1, 2010.

The Joint Commission: Medical Staff Standard MS.08.01.01-MS.08.01.03. 2010. Available at: http://www.jointcommission.org. Accessed February 1, 2010.

McNeil DE, Fordwood SR, Weaver CM, et al: Effects of training on suicide risk assessment. Psychiatr Serv 59:1462–1465, 2008

Scheiber SC, Kramer TS, Adamowski SE: Core Competencies for Psychiatric Practice: What Clinicians Need to Know (A Report of the American Board of Psychiatry and Neurology). Washington, DC, American Psychiatric Publishing, 2003

Simon RI: Suicide risk assessment: what is the standard of care? J Am Acad Psychiatry Law 30:340–344, 2002

Simon RI: Suicide risk: assessing the unpredictable, in The American Psychiatric Publishing Textbook of Suicide Assessment and Management. Edited by Simon RI, Hales RE. Washington, DC, American Psychiatric Publishing, 2006, pp 1–32

Simon RI: Suicide risk assessment forms: form over substance? J Am Acad Psychiatry Law 37:290–293, 2009

Simon RI, Shuman DW: Therapeutic risk management of clinical-legal dilemmas: should it be a core competency. J Am Acad Psychiatry Law 37:156–161, 2009

Sokolov G, Hilty DM, Leamon M, et al: Inpatient treatment and partial hospitalization, in The American Psychiatric Publishing Textbook of Suicide Assessment and Management. Edited by Simon RI, Hales RE. Washington, DC, American Psychiatric Publishing, 2006, pp 401–419

Sullivan GR, Bongar B: Psychological testing in suicide risk management, in The American Psychiatric Publishing Textbook of Suicide Assessment and Management. Edited by Simon RI, Hales RE. Washington, DC, American Psychiatric Publishing, 2006, pp 177–196

CHAPTER 13

Therapeutic Risk Management of the Patient at Risk for Suicide

Clinical-Legal Dilemmas

THE law has come to play a pervasive role in the practice of psychiatry (Simon 2009). The contours of the doctor-patient relationship are no longer defined solely by the psychiatrist and the patient. Courts, legislatures, and administrative agencies also shape the practice of psychiatry. Knowledge of the legal regulation of psychiatry that informs

Adapted from Simon RI, Shuman DW: "Therapeutic Risk Management of Clinical-Legal Dilemmas: Should It Be a Core Competency?" *Journal of the American Academy of Psychiatry and the Law* 35:156–161, 2009. © American Academy of Psychiatry and the Law. Reprinted with permission.

clinical practice is no longer optional for a psychiatrist. The requirements of the law must be integrated with best practices to achieve optimal therapeutic benefits. Effective management of the risks inherent in the practice of psychiatry in addition to the risks that external regulation generates is a reality of psychiatric practice.

Short of not seeing patients, there is nothing a psychiatrist can do that will reduce the risk of a lawsuit to zero. It is commonly understood that the goal of risk management is to reduce the likelihood of a successful malpractice suit or to maximize the success of a legal defense, if suit is brought.

Psychiatrists are frequently sued for patient suicide attempts and completions (see Figure 13–1). The treatment and management of suicidal patients present clinical-legal dilemmas that, if not appropriately managed, can harm the patient as well as expose the psychiatrist to malpractice liability.

Therapeutic risk management, a concept introduced here, assumes there is an optimal therapeutic accord to be found in each case, which demands a working knowledge of the law that regulates the practice of psychiatry, in addition to clinical competence. Successful resolution of clinical-legal dilemmas requires an understanding of the legal process that helps clinicians to provide good patient care and avoid unnecessary and counterproductive defensive practices. Most clinicians are not lawyers or forensic psychiatrists. But an understanding of how the law and psychiatry interact in clinical situations that occur frequently is essential. This is the essence of core competency. Good clinical practice and good laws are complementary (Wexler and Winick 1996).

Our Litigation Culture and Defensive Psychiatry

There are hundreds of medical malpractice suits pending in the United States at any given time (Meyer et al. 2010). These claims have an impact beyond the direct monetary costs (e.g., verdict or settlement, lawyers' fees, and lost income) and indirect costs (e.g., product or service redesign) associated with litigation. Malpractice suits also have a profound mental and emotional impact on physicians' personal and professional lives (Charles et al. 1985).

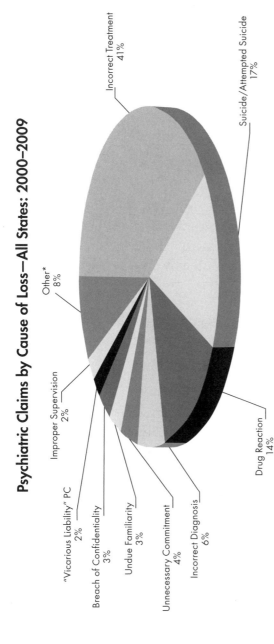

Psychiatric Claims by Cause of Loss—All States: 2000–2009

Incorrect Treatment 41%

Suicide/Attempted Suicide 17%

Drug Reaction 14%

Incorrect Diagnosis 6%

Unnecessary Commitment 4%

Undue Familiarity 3%

Breach of Confidentiality 3%

"Vicarious Liability" PC 2%

Improper Supervision 2%

Other* 8%

*Other: libel/slander, fen-phen, third party (e.g., parents), forensic, other/not specific, administrative, lack of informed consent, Tarasoff, none, abandonment, boundary violation, premises liability

The "cause of loss" represents the main allegation made in the claim or lawsuit. In almost all lawsuits multiple allegations of negligence are asserted. These data are collected based on the chief allegation or complaint. Thus, the category of "incorrect treatment" may be alleged in a lawsuit based on a patient suicide, but the main or chief allegation/complaint is stated as "incorrect treatment." Suicide and attempted suicide is the most frequently identifiable cause of loss. The "drug reaction" category used here encompasses all types of drug/medication misadventures, including errors in prescribing, adverse reactions to medications, mismanagement of a patient's medication regime, or other unanticipated outcomes related to medication use.

FIGURE 13–1.   Psychiatric claims by cause of loss—all states: 2000–2009.

Source.   The Psychiatrists' Program, managed by Professional Risk Management Services, Inc.

In one study, researchers compared physicians who were sued with physicians who were not sued. The physicians who were sued reported that they were significantly more likely to stop seeing certain patients, consider an early retirement, and discourage their children from entering a medical career. Patient suicides are among the most traumatic events in a psychiatrist's professional life (Gitlin 2006). Unfortunately, the current litigation climate encourages defensive practices that may neither protect the psychiatrist nor benefit the patient.

Defensive practices are intended to help the psychiatrist avoid a successful malpractice suit or provide a legal defense if sued. Defensive practices can be categorized as preemptive or avoidant and further subclassified as appropriate or inappropriate. Because a malpractice suit may follow a suicide attempt or completed suicide, the psychiatrist may utilize defensive practices that interfere with adequate treatment of patients at risk for suicide. For example, hospitalizing a patient at moderate risk for suicide is an inappropriate, preemptive defensive reaction when the patient can be safely treated as an outpatient. In fact, many patients assessed at moderate risk of suicide are treated as outpatients (Simon 2004).

Inappropriate, avoidant defensive practices cause the psychiatrist to forgo necessary treatments or procedures. An example is the psychiatrist who fails to treat a compliant suicidal schizophrenic patient with clozapine, a drug shown to reduce suicide attempts in schizophrenic patients, for fear of a lawsuit, if agranulocytosis develops. It is a potentially lethal side effect that occurs in less than 1% of patients (Alvir et al. 1993; Meltzer et al. 2003). Instead of avoidant defensive practices, good clinical care is the best risk management. Good clinical care requires the clinician to obtain the patient's or substitute decision-maker's informed consent for the drug and to carefully monitor the patient.

An example of an appropriate defensive measure that benefits both the psychiatrist and the patient is careful documentation of suicide risk assessments. In the event of a claim, it is also an important risk management tool demonstrating that suicide risk assessments were competently performed. Most appropriate avoidance risk management practices are inseparable from good clinical care.

When defensive practices direct rather than support clinical decision making, the outcome can be harmful to patient care, to the doctor-patient relationship, and to the professional integrity of the practitioner.

For example, psychiatry residents often have a fearful reaction to lawyers and lawsuits that can impair their clinical decision making. Paradoxically, inappropriate defensive practices, often the result of clinical-legal misunderstandings gone awry, can invite a lawsuit. The goal of therapeutic risk management is to effectively address clinical-legal dilemmas, while maintaining the integrity of the patient's treatment. The royal road to therapeutic risk management passes through good patient care. It does not veer off into a detour of self-defensive practices.

The Suicidal Patient: A Paradigm for Therapeutic Risk Management

It is a clinical axiom that there are two kinds of psychiatrists—those who have had patients complete suicide and those who will. Most psychiatrists in clinical practice currently treat one or more patients at risk for suicide. Patient suicides are an unavoidable occupational hazard of psychiatric practice. Completed suicide and suicide attempts are the most frequent claims of loss in psychiatric malpractice cases. Suicidal patients frequently challenge the clinician with thorny clinical-legal dilemmas.

Suicide risk assessment is a core competency that psychiatrists must possess, informing the treatment and management of all patients (Scheiber et al. 2003). A core competency is defined as "[t]hose skills and abilities that are central to, or 'at the core' of a given field" (Scheiber et al. 2003, p. 65). In patients at suicide risk, the standard of care requires that the psychiatrist perform reasonable suicide risk assessments (Simon 2003; Simon and Shuman 2006). Yet review of hospital and outpatient psychiatric records rarely reveals adequate documentation of suicide risk assessments, raising questions about whether such assessments were actually performed (Simon 2004).

Therapeutic risk management affirms the clinician's role in the treatment of the suicidal patient. It requires a working knowledge of the legal regulation of psychiatry that informs appropriate clinical management of legal issues frequently arising with high-risk suicidal patients. For example, clinical-legal issues often involve confidentiality; competency/incompetency; the right to treatment; informed consent; freedom of movement (least restrictive alternative); seclusion and restraint; involuntary treatment (medication, hospitalization); and electroconvulsive therapy (ECT).

Therapeutic risk management is inherently good clinical care. It supports the patient's treatment and the therapeutic alliance. The pervasive ethic is beneficence and, "First do no harm." Therapeutic risk management avoids defensive practices of dubious benefit that, paradoxically, can invite a malpractice suit. Moreover, an unduly defensive mindset can distract the clinician from providing good patient care (Simon 1985).

Case Example[1]

A 37-year-old accountant with severe depression, persistent suicidal ideation, and a plan to jump from a nearby bridge is admitted to a psychiatric unit. The patient's depression is resistant to medications. A psychiatric consultation is obtained in which the consultant recommends ECT. The patient possesses the mental capacity to consent to ECT. The psychiatrist, however, is concerned about being sued, especially if memory impairment occurs. The psychiatrist decides to obtain permission for ECT from the family. The patient pleads for ECT, "I can't stand the pain much longer." The ECT is delayed because of the family's ambivalence about the treatment. The patient attempts suicide by hanging. He is rescued by the inpatient staff and survives, but with resulting severe brain damage. On behalf of the patient, the patient's family files a lawsuit against the psychiatrist and the hospital for "negligent treatment."

Case Commentary

The case above demonstrates how deviant defensive practices can interfere with the treatment of a patient at very high risk for suicide, resulting in a suicide attempt. There is no authority that equates severe depression with incompetence in all cases or prohibits a patient with severe depression from consenting to the administration of ECT. Consent of family members of a competent patient was not required for ECT. Lawsuits involving ECT are relatively rare (Simon 2004). No increase in malpractice insurance premium is attached to performing ECT. A psychiatrist is more likely to be sued for failing to provide timely

---

[1]The case examples in this chapter are an amalgam of disguised, litigated, and clinical cases.

ECT for a severely depressed patient who is at acute, high risk for suicide, for whom mainstay treatments have failed (Gitlin 2006).

Therapeutic Risk Management: Maintaining the Locus of Attention on Patient Care

Negligence is a system for imposing liability based on an assessment of the reasonableness of a person's actions judged prospectively. Justice Benjamin Cardozo, the author of *Palsgraf v. Long Island R.R.* (1928), a seminal decision in the law of torts, articulated the relationship ascribed between risk and duties we owe to others: "The risk reasonably to be perceived defines the duty to be obeyed, and risk imports relation; it is risk to another or to others within the range of apprehension. The range of reasonable apprehension is at times a question for the court, and at times, if varying inferences are possible, a question for the jury." Risk management attempts to provide that guidance through measures to diminish loss. Risk management for the suicidal patient addresses the potential harms arising from his or her mental disorder as well as from treatment interventions or omissions.

In therapeutic risk management, the locus of attention is on the suicidal patient. It is a part of the clinical process that supports good patient care. In malpractice risk management, the locus of attention is primarily on the psychiatrist, though it is not intended to harm the patient. For example, liability-based risk management principles, derived from lessons learned in studying malpractice claims and litigation, provide important practical pointers, often best practices, for managing liability risk in the treatment of suicidal patients. The following are examples of the bases for claims in the context of suicide attempts or completed suicides (Psychiatrists' Purchasing Group 2002):

- Failure to provide proper assessment and management in high-volume patient settings
- Failure to construct a comprehensive treatment plan
- Failure to perform comprehensive suicide risk assessments
- Failure to document suicide risk assessments
- Failure to obtain past treatment records

- Failure to hospitalize
- Failure to make a rational diagnosis on the basis of the history and evaluation

There is a case-specific, dynamic tension between a psychiatrist's therapeutic and malpractice locus of attention, as illustrated in all the case examples. Clinical-legal dilemmas, unless properly managed, can shift the locus of attention toward liability risk management. The clinician must determine where the appropriate locus of attention should be at any given time and in any clinical circumstance. Both foci are necessary in informing risk management. When a clinical-legal dilemma shifts the clinician's locus of attention away from patient care to malpractice risk management, the potential for inappropriate defensive practice increases.

In clinical practice, situations arise in which the psychiatrist's locus of attention must necessarily be on malpractice prevention, though not to the detriment of patient care. The clinician's locus of attention on malpractice risk management is appropriate, for example, when a depressed suicidal patient who does not meet the criteria for involuntary hospitalization, leaves the hospital against medical advice (AMA). Careful documentation of discussions that take place with the patient regarding the risks of premature discharge and the need for continued treatment is necessary. Merely having the patient sign an AMA form is insufficient (Gerbasi and Simon 2003). This procedure is necessary for the sole protection of the psychiatrist and the hospital against a malpractice suit, even though a therapeutic outcome may still be possible.

Case Example

A psychiatrist is conducting medication management of a patient assessed at chronic, high risk for suicide. He learns from the psychotherapist that their patient has recently purchased a handgun. The patient's risk has changed from chronic to acute, high risk because of the gun purchase. Fearing a malpractice suit, the psychiatrist considers calling the police or notifying the patient's father without the patient's permission or certifying the patient for involuntary hospitalization.

The psychiatrist, who is losing sleep worrying about the patient, obtains a psychiatric consultation. The consultant recommends that the patient's purchase of a handgun be addressed immediately as a treatment issue. Psychiatric hospitalization still remains an option. The consultant believes that asking the patient to relinquish the handgun to a responsible third party will be a test of the therapeutic alliance. The psychiatrist and the psychotherapist affirm their commitment to the patient's treatment but inform the patient that treatment cannot continue if the patient keeps the gun. The patient acquiesces, turning the handgun over to her father. Thus, stringent measures such as involuntary hospitalization are temporarily avoided, but would have been necessary if the treatment approach failed.

The psychiatrist carefully documents the decision-making process, a good clinical practice and sound malpractice risk management. The psychiatrist requests a written report from the consultant. Therapeutic risk management maintains the locus of attention on patient care, thus avoiding disruption of the patient's treatment. The therapeutic alliance with the patient is strengthened, thus decreasing the suicide risk.

Case Commentary

The case example above illustrates how therapeutic risk management can shift the locus of attention back to the patient and away from unnecessary defensive actions (e.g., calling the police or breaching confidentiality) that could disrupt the patient's treatment and increase suicide risk. When clinical-legal dilemmas arise in split-treatment arrangements, the clinician's therapeutic risk management locus may be difficult to maintain because of limitations on time and frequency of visits. Inappropriate defensive practices can become "stealth" suicide risk factors.

A clinician's negative reaction to patients at risk for suicide may include anger, hate, despair, frustration, and hopelessness (Maltsberger and Buie 1974). The clinician may use defensive reaction formation to deny hostile feelings toward the suicidal patient who threatens the clinician's competence and raises the fear of a lawsuit (Gabbard 1995). Destructive defensive measures such as premature discharge abandon the patient and increase suicide risk. Consultation can restore the clinician's equanimity, thus avoiding potential countertherapeutic defensive reactions. The clinician should "never worry alone" (T.G. Gutheil, personal communication, June 2008).

Good Clinical Care:
Is It Good Enough?

Good clinical care, in most instances, provides solid risk management, although risk management is not usually the primary concern. For example, when possible, speaking with family members about a suicidal patient is both good clinical care and good risk management. Patients at high risk for suicide often inform a family member about suicide ideation, intent, or plan, but do not tell the clinician (Simon 2006).

Good clinical care, however, is not synonymous with therapeutic risk management. Although good clinical care is necessary, it may not be sufficient in reducing malpractice risk. Good clinical care can deteriorate into inappropriate defensive practices when clinicians are confronted by complex clinical-legal issues. As noted earlier, therapeutic risk management additionally applies an understanding of the legal regulation of psychiatry to clinical-legal issues that arise in the patient's treatment. For example, good clinical care respects the suicidal patient's right to refuse necessary treatment. Employing best practice, the clinician attempts to build a therapeutic alliance with the patient, which is made a more difficult task in the era of brief psychiatric hospitalization of serious ill patients. An exception, however, allows the psychiatrist to treat the high-risk suicidal patient in an emergency. The emergency exception is embodied in case law in some states and in statutory law in others, with a definition of what constitutes an emergency that varies from state to state (Simon and Shuman 2009). Under the common law, as well as statutory codifications, informed consent has not been required when an "emergency of such gravity and urgency exists that it is impractical to obtain the patient's consent" (*Wright v. Johns Hopkins Health Systems Corp.* 1999).

The legal standard of care does not require the psychiatrist to adhere to best practices, or even to provide good clinical care to the patient. The law articulating the standard of care, both in the legislative and judicial voices, varies among the states from customary practice to the practice of the reasonable, prudent practitioner (Simon and Shuman 2007). Although the provision of good clinical care and a working understanding of clinical-legal management cannot construct an impenetrable barrier against a malpractice suit, it provides an important strategic option.

Case Example

A 63-year-old retired attorney is admitted to a psychiatric inpatient unit with a diagnosis of major depression, single-episode, severe, with psychotic features. Prominent symptoms include intense suicidal ideation, ideas of reference, and insomnia and anxiety. Mild cognitive impairment is also noted. Because the patient is an attorney, the unit staff requests that the patient sign and honor a suicide prevention contract. The patient, however, refuses to sign. Dr. Wright does not rely on "no harm" contracts. The psychiatrist practices therapeutic risk management. She maintains the locus of attention on the patient, performing systematic suicide assessments that inform continuing treatment and safety management. Dr. Wright does not use suicide risk assessment forms, but instead employs a risk assessment approach based on her education, training, clinical experience, and a familiarity with the current professional literature. Her understanding of the standard of care for suicide risk assessment is that it encompasses a range of reasonable assessment methods (Simon and Shuman 2006).

Dr. Wright's initial suicide risk assessment determines that the patient is at acute, high risk for suicide. The patient is placed on one-to-one visual observation. He threatens to sue the staff for "spying" and restricting his freedom. Dr. Wright manages the threat of litigation as a treatment-related issue to be discussed with the patient, instead of reacting defensively. Clinical decision-making rationale is documented. Although everything of significance cannot be documented, Dr. Wright follows standard practice in documenting important clinical assessments and interventions. The record becomes an active clinical tool that facilitates continuity of the patient's care, not just an inert document aimed at lowering liability risk. She treats the patient, not the chart. Dr. Wright expects that in a lawsuit, plaintiff's counsel will make the argument in court that what was not documented was not done.

The psychiatrist tries to build a therapeutic alliance with the patient. The patient, who has a daughter similar in age to the psychiatrist, responds positively, but continues to complain bitterly about the staff. The patient withholds permission for the psychiatrist or staff to call his wife or daughter. However, Dr. Wright tells the patient that she would like to listen to family members who call but would do so without having to disclose confidences. He consents. The patient refuses to take medications and wants to leave the hospital against medical advice. Because he was admitted as a conditional voluntary admission, he can be held for 72 hours, if he is deemed a danger to himself or others.

The patient calls his attorney, demanding a habeas corpus hearing. He again threatens Dr. Wright with a lawsuit. She consults the in-hospital counsel to minimize its potential interference with the patient's treatment. The hospital attorney explains the legal issues relating to habeas corpus and opines that it is unlikely a judge would order the release of the patient. A psychiatric consultation is also obtained. The psychiatric consultant supports Dr. Wright's current treatment plan.

Dr. Wright informs the patient that he is seriously ill and in critical need of treatment. If necessary, she will certify the patient for involuntary hospitalization to ensure that he receives urgent treatment and remains safe. She continues the process of documenting her decision-making rationale. Dr. Wright understands the importance of documenting "why," not just "what." She decides to treat the patient only with his consent, although an emergency exception to consent could be justified. Dr. Wright works at developing a therapeutic alliance. The patient has cognitive deficits, but he still has the mental capacity to give consent. Dr. Wright calls the patient's wife for more information, after the patient provides a written authorization for release of information. The patient settles down and agrees to stay. He accepts treatment and improves.

Case Commentary

In the case example above, therapeutic risk management supports the treatment provided the patient. Dr. Wright keeps her locus of attention on patient care. She is neither intimidated in treating a potentially litigious patient nor drawn into self-defeating defensive actions. Documented systematic suicide risk assessments are performed that direct treatment (Simon 2003). The record does not contain the all too familiar "No SI, HI, CFS" (no suicidal ideation, homicidal ideation, contracts for safety). Dr. Wright knows that documentation of substandard risk assessments is worse than no documentation. No reliance is placed on safety contracts. She knows that no scientific evidence exists to prove that safety contracts diminish or eliminate suicide risk (Garvey et al. 2009; Stanford et al. 1994).

Dr. Wright does not rely on risk assessment forms, especially checklists, in conducting suicide risk assessment. She knows that checklists and other suicide risk forms cannot encompass all the unique, individual, suicide risk factors presented by the patient (Simon 2009). Moreover "risk factors" are often included in checklists for which no evidence-based studies exist. No checklist can be complete. In suicide cases in litigation, a plaintiff's attorney will seize on an invariable omission of relevant risk factors from the stock checklist used to assess the patient.

Dr. Wright consults with the hospital attorney to clarify the habeas corpus issue in order to minimize its potential interference with the patient's treatment. A psychiatric consultation supports her clinical management of the patient, providing a "biopsy" of the standard of care. She does not "worry alone." Dr. Wright's reasons for obtaining psychiatric and legal consultations are twofold: to assure good clinical care and, secondarily, to confirm that the patient's treatment and management meet the standard of care.

Dr. Wright confronts the patient with involuntary hospitalization in a clinically supportive manner, but nonetheless is decisive and firm. She possesses a clinically liberating knowledge of the legal regulation of psychiatry. For example, Dr. Wright understands that an emergency exception to voluntary consent to treatment is available, but decides not to invoke it. Instead, consent to treatment is initially managed as a treatment issue. She knows that the determination of mental capacity is a reasoned clinical judgment. Dr. Wright concludes that her patient can provide competent consent to treatment, despite mild cognitive impairment. She distinguishes between mental capacity and competency, the latter being a judicial determination.

Dr. Wright understands the substantive and procedural criteria for involuntary hospitalization in her state and the emergency exceptions to maintaining confidentiality. She keeps a copy of the commitment statute readily available and is comfortable handling clinical-legal situations. She is not dislodged from her clinical role with the patient, despite his threat of a lawsuit. Dr. Wright also carries good professional liability insurance.

Conclusion

A tension can arise between what the law demands and what good clinical care requires. Accepting that tension as a limitation on clinical practice is a self-fulfilling prophecy that ill serves psychiatrists and their patients. What the law requires is often the subject of misinformation and confusion. An often unintended consequence is inappropriate defensive practices.

It is a reality that law plays a pervasive role in psychiatric practice. A working knowledge of how the law and psychiatry interact in clinical-legal situations that occur frequently is essential. Therapeutic risk management should be a core competency in psychiatry that demands an awareness of that dynamic tension between psychiatry and the law and an acceptance of the responsibility to find an optimal balance in the care of the patient.

KEY CLINICAL CONCEPTS

- The royal road to therapeutic risk management passes through good patient care, not veering off into a detour of self-defeating defensive practices.

- Therapeutic risk management of clinical-legal dilemmas achieves an optimal alignment between clinical competence and an understanding of legal issues applicable to psychiatric practice.

- Understanding how psychiatry and law interact in clinical situations that occur frequently is essential to effective care of the suicidal patient.

- Successful management of clinical-legal dilemmas avoids unnecessary, counterproductive defensive practices.

- Defensive practices can be categorized as preemptive or avoidant, and further subclassified as appropriate or inappropriate.

References

Alvir JM, Lieberman JA, Safferman AZ, et al: Clozapine-induced agranulocytosis. Incidence and risk factors in the United States. N Engl J Med 329:162–167, 1993

Charles SC, Wilbert JR, Franke KJ: Sued and nonsued physicians' self-reported reactions to malpractice litigation. Am J Psychiatry 142:437–440, 1985

Gabbard GO, Lester EF: Boundaries and Boundary Violations in Psychoanalysis. New York, Basic Books, 1995

Garvey KA, Penn JV, Campbell AL, et al: Contracting for safety with patients: clinical practice and forensic implications. J Am Acad Psychiatry Law 37:363–370, 2009

Gerbasi JB, Simon RI: When patients leave the hospital against medical advice: patients' rights and psychiatrists' duties. Harv Rev Psychiatry 11:333–343, 2003

Gitlin M: Psychiatrist reactions to suicide, in The American Psychiatric Publishing Textbook of Suicide Assessment and Management. Edited by Simon RI, Hales RE. Washington, DC, American Psychiatric Publishing, 2006, pp 477–492

Maltsberger JT, Buie DC: Countertransference hate in the treatment of suicidal patients. Arch Gen Psychiatry 30:625–633, 1974

Meltzer HY, Alphs L, Green AI, et al: Clozapine treatment for suicidality in schizophrenia: International Suicide Intervention Trial (InterSePT). Arch Gen Psychiatry 60:82–91, 2003

Meyer DJ, Simon RI, Shuman DW: Psychiatric malpractice and the standard of care, in The American Psychiatric Publishing Textbook of Forensic Psychiatry, 2nd Edition. Edited by Simon RI, Gold LH. Washington, DC, American Psychiatric Publishing, 2010, pp 207–226

Palsgraf v Long Island R.R., 16 N.E. 99 (NY 1928)

Psychiatrists' Purchasing Group, Component Workshop: Risk Management Issues in Psychiatric Practice. Presented at the 155th annual meeting of the American Psychiatric Association, Philadelphia, PA, May 20, 2002

Scheiber SC, Kramer TS, Adamowski SE: Core Competencies for Psychiatric Practice: What Clinicians Need to Know (A Report of the American Board of Psychiatry and Neurology). Washington, DC, American Psychiatric Publishing, 2003

Simon RI: Coping strategies for the defensive psychiatrist. Med Law 4:551–561, 1985

Simon RI: Suicide risk assessment: what is the standard of care? J Am Acad Psychiatry Law 31:65–67, 2003

Simon RI: Assessing and Managing Suicide Risk: Guidelines for Clinically Based Risk Management. Washington, DC, American Psychiatric Publishing, 2004, pp 39, 142, 153

Simon RI: Suicide risk assessment: assessing the unpredictable, in The American Psychiatric Publishing Textbook of Suicide Assessment and Management. Edited by Simon RI, Hales RE. Washington, DC, American Psychiatric Publishing, 2006, pp 1–32

Simon RI: Suicide risk assessment forms: form over substance? J Am Acad Psychiatry Law 37:290–293, 2009

Simon RI, Shuman DW: The standard of care in suicide risk assessment: an elusive concept. CNS Spectr 11:442–445, 2006

Simon RI, Shuman DW: Clinical Manual of Psychiatry and Law. Washington, DC, American Psychiatric Publishing, 2007, p 6

Simon RI, Shuman DW: Clinical-legal issues of psychiatry, in Comprehensive Textbook of Psychiatry, 8th Edition. Edited by Sadock BJ, Sadock VA. Philadelphia, PA, Lippincott Williams & Williams, 2009, pp 4427–4438

Stanford EJ, Goetz RR, Bloom JD: The no harm contract in the emergency assessment of suicide risk. J Clin Psychiatry 55:344–348, 1994

Wexler DB, Winick BJ: Essays in Therapeutic Jurisprudence. Durham, NC, Carolina Academic Press, 1991

Wexler DB, Winick BJ: Law in a Therapeutic Key: Developments in Therapeutic Jurisprudence. Durham, NC, Carolina Academic Press, 1996

Wright v. Johns Hopkins Health Systems Corp., 728 A.2d 166 (Md 1999)

Suicide Risk Assessment Self-Test

The 50-item true-false self-test is a teaching instrument designed to enhance clinician suicide risk assessment. Scoring is by and for the test-taker. The questions are selected from material in this book and from referenced sources.

Questions

1. The purpose of suicide risk assessment is to inform patient treatment and management, not the prediction of suicide.

   ❒ True
   ❒ False

2. Eating disorders have the highest standard mortality ratio (SMR)[1] for suicide.

   ❒ True
   ❒ False

---

[1]SMR is a measure of the relative risk of suicide for a particular psychiatric disorder compared with the expected rate in the general population.

3. Of the three personality disorder clusters, Cluster C is most frequently associated with suicide.

    ❐ True
    ❐ False

4. The numbers of comorbid disorders, not the types of disorders, significantly increase suicide risk.

    ❐ True
    ❐ False

5. Most evidence-based suicide risk and protective factors are derived from community-based psychological autopsy studies.

    ❐ True
    ❐ False

6. The increased risk of a firearm suicide occurs within 1 week after purchase of a handgun.

    ❐ True
    ❐ False

7. Documented, competent suicide risk assessments are a rarity.

    ❐ True
    ❐ False

8. There are a number of acceptable methods for conducting suicide risk assessments.

    ❐ True
    ❐ False

9. Suicide prevention contracts are important in the management of the patient with borderline disorder at risk for suicide.

    ❐ True
    ❐ False

10. Studies have shown that religious affiliation is a protective factor against suicide.

    ❐ True
    ❐ False

11. The legal standard of care requires that suicide risk assessments be reasonable.

    ❏ True
    ❏ False

12. Lithium and clozapine, respectively, reduce suicide attempts in patients with bipolar disorder and schizophrenia.

    ❏ True
    ❏ False

13. A high educational level is a protective factor against suicide.

    ❏ True
    ❏ False

14. The standard mortality ratio (SMR) is elevated for all psychiatric disorders, including mental retardation.

    ❏ True
    ❏ False

15. Approximately 25% of suicidal patients do not admit to suicidal ideation but do tell their families.

    ❏ True
    ❏ False

16. Among individuals attempting suicide, 90% of unplanned and 60% of planned suicide attempts occur within 1 year of suicide ideation onset.

    ❏ True
    ❏ False

17. Living with a child under age 18 years is a protective factor against suicide.

    ❏ True
    ❏ False

18. Short-term suicide risk factors are useful in assessing the likelihood of a suicide attempt within 24–48 hours.

    ❏ True
    ❏ False

19. The risk of suicide is highest during the first year following a suicide attempt.

    ❐ True
    ❐ False

20. Among patients who have made a suicide attempt, 30% eventually complete suicide.

    ❐ True
    ❐ False

21. Prior suicide attempts and hopelessness are powerful clinical "predictors" of completed suicide.

    ❐ True
    ❐ False

22. In adolescents, there is little evidence that "contagion effects" can lead to suicidal behaviors following personal contact with a suicide.

    ❐ True
    ❐ False

23. In the Copenhagen Adoption Study, biological relatives of adoptees who completed suicide did not have an increase in suicide as compared with biological relatives of matched adoptees who did not complete suicide.

    ❐ True
    ❐ False

24. Melancholic depression is associated with increased suicide risk as compared with depression without melancholic features.

    ❐ True
    ❐ False

25. Patients with psychotic disorders are not at increased risk of suicide compared with nonpsychotic patients.

    ❐ True
    ❐ False

26. Evidence-based suicide risk factors are derived from systematic reviews as well as cohort and case-control studies.

    ❐ True
    ❐ False

27. Violent threats or behaviors toward others are suicide risk factors.

    ❐ True
    ❐ False

28. The preferred study designs for determining suicide risk are cohort and case-control studies.

    ❐ True
    ❐ False

29. Following inpatient discharge, the risk of suicide is highest during the first week.

    ❐ True
    ❐ False

30. The absolute risk of suicide in patients with bipolar disorder is 193 per 100,000. This means that 99,807 patients with bipolar disorder will not commit suicide.

    ❐ True
    ❐ False

31. No suicide risk assessment method has been tested for reliability and validity.

    ❐ True
    ❐ False

32. General suicide risk factors as compared with individual risk factors are derived from community-based psychological autopsies in addition to cohort and case-control studies.

    ❐ True
    ❐ False

33. Individual suicide risk factors tend to be idiosyncratic and not essential to suicide risk assessment.

   ❏ True
   ❏ False

34. Suicidal patients often display recurrent prodromal suicide risk factors before attempting or completing suicide.

   ❏ True
   ❏ False

35. The severity of mental illness can nullify protective factors against suicide attempts.

   ❏ True
   ❏ False

36. Patients with personality disorders are not at increased risk of suicide, unless comorbid with an Axis I psychiatric disorder.

   ❏ True
   ❏ False

37. Admission to a psychiatric inpatient unit or hospital is not, by itself, a significant suicide risk factor.

   ❏ True
   ❏ False

38. A single suicide risk factor does not have sufficient statistical power on which to base an assessment.

   ❏ True
   ❏ False

39. Patients who attempt or complete suicide are more impulsive than the general population.

   ❏ True
   ❏ False

40. No method of suicide risk assessment can identify who will commit suicide (sensitivity) and who will not (specificity).

    ❐ True
    ❐ False

41. The standard of care requires that assessment forms or checklists accompany suicide risk assessments.

    ❐ True
    ❐ False

42. The therapeutic alliance cannot be considered a protective factor, because it varies from patient to patient or unpredictably with individual patients.

    ❐ True
    ❐ False

43. When lethal means to complete suicide are less available, rates of suicide by lethal methods decline.

    ❐ True
    ❐ False

44. Before discharging an inpatient at low to moderate risk for suicide who has guns at home, the standard of care requires that the clinician receive a callback from a designated third-party, confirming that the guns have been removed and secured according to a prearranged plan.

    ❐ True
    ❐ False

45. Sudden improvement in a high-risk suicidal patient requires an immediate increase in observational level.

    ❐ True
    ❐ False

46. Observational data (behavioral suicide risk factors) can assist in the early identification of the guarded suicidal patient.

    ❐ True
    ❐ False

47. Statutory commitment laws require the clinician to involuntarily hospitalize the acute, high-risk suicidal patient.

    ❐ True
    ❐ False

48. Actuarial analysis of suicide risk identifies specific, treatable risk and modifiable protective factors.

    ❐ True
    ❐ False

49. Suicide risk increases with the total number of risk factors, providing a quasi-quantitative dimension to suicide risk assessment.

    ❐ True
    ❐ False

50. A frequent flaw of suicide risk assessment forms is the omission of protective factors.

    ❐ True
    ❐ False

Answers

1. True

2. True

3. False: correct answer is—Cluster B

4. True

5. False: correct answer is—also cohort and case-control studies

6. True

7. True

8. True

9. False: correct answer is—no evidence that suicide prevention contracts prevent suicide

10. True

11. True

12. True

13. False: correct answer is—no evidence to support statement

14. False: correct answer is—no elevated suicide risk in mental retardation

15. True

16. True

17. True

18. False: correct answer is—no evidence-based, short-term suicide risk factors

19. True

20. False: correct answer is—10%–15%

21. True

22. False: correct answer is—"contagion effects" increase suicide risk in adolescents

23. False: correct answer is—sixfold increase in suicide in biological relatives of adoptee studies

24. True

25. False: correct answer is—suicide risk in psychiatric patient is two times greater

26. True

27. True

28. True

29. True

30. True

31. True

32. True

33. False: correct answer is—individual suicide risk factors are essential and must be assessed.

34. True

35. True

36. False: correct answer is—personality disorders, without comorbidity, place patients at increased risk of suicide

37. False: correct answer is—a high risk factor

38. True

39. True

40. True

41. False: correct answer is—no such requirement exists

42. False: correct answer is—though variable, the therapeutic alliance is a key protective factor

43. True

44. True

45. False: correct answer is—obtain corroborative evidence of improvement (e.g., from family, staff, observed behaviors)

46. True

47. False: correct answer is—involuntary hospitalization is a clinical decision; commitment laws are only permissive

48. False: correct answer is—only clinical assessment identifies specific risk and protective factors

49. True

50. True

Sources

Practice guideline for the assessment and treatment of patients with suicidal behaviors. Am J Psychiatry 160 (11 suppl):1–60, 2003

Simon RI: Assessing and Managing Suicide Risk: Guidelines for Clinically Based Risk Management. Washington, DC, American Psychiatric Publishing, 2004

Simon RI, Hales RE (eds): The American Psychiatric Publishing Textbook of Suicide Assessment and Management. Washington, DC, American Psychiatric Publishing, 2006

Index

*Page numbers printed in **boldface** type refer to tables or figures.*